Handbook of
Recurrent Pregnancy Loss

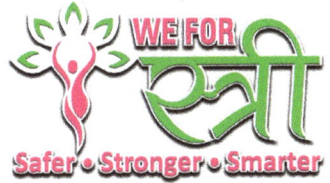

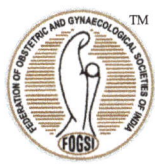

Federation of Obstetric and Gynaecological Societies of India (FOGSI)

Handbook of
Recurrent Pregnancy Loss

Series Editors

Nandita Palshetkar
MD FCPS FICOG FRCOG(UK)
President of FOGSI 2019
Scientific Director, Bloom IVF
Professor of Obstetrics and Gynecology
Dr DY Patil Medical College, Hospital and
Research Centre
Navi Mumbai, Maharashtra, India

Rohan Palshetkar
MS(Obs/Gyne) FRM
ART Consultant and Endoscopic Surgeon
Associate Professor
DY Patil Medical College
Unit Head
DY Patil Bloom IVF
Navi Mumbai, Maharashtra, India

Editors

Jayam Kannan
MD DGO FICOG
Vice-President, FOGSI 2018
Emeritus Professor
Tamil Nadu Dr MGR Medical University
Director
Garbba Rakshambigai Fertility Centre
Chennai, Tamil Nadu, India

Hrishikesh D Pai
MD FCPS FICOG MSc(USA) FRCOG
Scientific Director, Bloom IVF
Secretary General, FOGSI 2015-17
Gynecologist and Head of IVF Unit
Lilavati Hospital
Mumbai, Maharashtra, India

Charmila Ayyavoo
MD DGO DFP FICOG PGDCR
Director, Aditi Hospital and Parvathy Ayyavoo Fertility Centre, Trichy
Consultant, Southern Railway Hospital, Trichy
Secretary, Trichy OG Society 2012-13
Chairperson, Clinical Research Committee, FOGSI 2016-18
President, Menstrual Hygiene Management Consortium
Chennai, Tamil Nadu, India

Foreword
Nandita Palshetkar

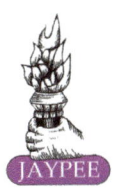

JAYPEE BROTHERS MEDICAL PUBLISHERS
The Health Sciences Publisher
New Delhi | London

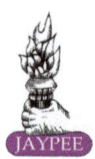 **Jaypee Brothers Medical Publishers (P) Ltd.**

Headquarters
Jaypee Brothers Medical Publishers (P) Ltd
4838/24, Ansari Road, Daryaganj
New Delhi 110 002, India
Phone: +91-11-43574357
Fax: +91-11-43574314
E-mail: jaypee@jaypeebrothers.com

Overseas Office
JP Medical Ltd
83 Victoria Street, London
SW1H 0HW (UK)
Phone: +44 20 3170 8910
Fax: +44 (0)20 3008 6180
E-mail: info@jpmedpub.com

Website: www.jaypeebrothers.com
Website: www.jaypeedigital.com

© 2020, Jaypee Brothers Medical Publishers

The views and opinions expressed in this book are solely those of the original contributor(s)/author(s) and do not necessarily represent those of editor(s) of the book.

All rights reserved. No part of this publication may be reproduced, stored or transmitted in any form or by any means, electronic, mechanical, photocopying, recording or otherwise, without the prior permission in writing of the publishers.

All brand names and product names used in this book are trade names, service marks, trademarks or registered trademarks of their respective owners. The publisher is not associated with any product or vendor mentioned in this book.

Medical knowledge and practice change constantly. This book is designed to provide accurate, authoritative information about the subject matter in question. However, readers are advised to check the most current information available on procedures included and check information from the manufacturer of each product to be administered, to verify the recommended dose, formula, method and duration of administration, adverse effects and contraindications. It is the responsibility of the practitioner to take all appropriate safety precautions. Neither the publisher nor the author(s)/editor(s) assume any liability for any injury and/or damage to persons or property arising from or related to use of material in this book.

This book is sold on the understanding that the publisher is not engaged in providing professional medical services. If such advice or services are required, the services of a competent medical professional should be sought.

Every effort has been made where necessary to contact holders of copyright to obtain permission to reproduce copyright material. If any have been inadvertently overlooked, the publisher will be pleased to make the necessary arrangements at the first opportunity. The **CD/DVD-ROM** (if any) provided in the sealed envelope with this book is complimentary and free of cost. **Not meant for sale.**

Inquiries for bulk sales may be solicited at: jaypee@jaypeebrothers.com

Handbook of Recurrent Pregnancy Loss

First Edition: 2020
ISBN: 978-93-89188-71-4

Dedicated to
All fellow FOGSIANs, our family and friends.

Dedicated to

Office Bearers of Team FOGSI 2019

President	Dr Nandita Palshetkar
Secretary General	Dr Jaydeep Tank
Vice President (West Zone)	Dr Rajendrasingh Pardeshi
Vice President (West Zone)	Dr Haresh Doshi
Vice President (North Zone)	Dr Sudha Prasad
Vice President (East Zone)	Dr Rajat Mohanty
Vice President (South Zone)	Dr Aswath Kumar
Deputy Secretary General	Dr Madhuri Patel
Treasurer	Dr Suvarna Khadilkar
Joint Treasurer	Dr Parikshit Tank
Joint Secretary	Dr Ameya Purandare
Immediate Past President	Dr Jaideep Malhotra
President Elect	Dr Alpesh Gandhi

Chairpersons of the Committees

Adolescent Health	Dr Girish Mane
Chnical Research	Dr Meena Samant
Endocrinology	Dr Pratik Tambe
Endometriosis	Dr Kuldeep Jain
Endoscopic Surgery	Dr B Ramesh
Ethics and Medicolegal	Dr Geetendra Sharma
Family Welfare	Dr Shobha Gudi
Food Drugs Medico Surgical Equipment	Dr Vidya Thobbi
Genetics and Fetal Medicine	Dr Mandakini Pradhan
HIV/AIDS	Dr Mrutyunjay Mohapatra
Imaging Science	Dr Meenu Agarwal
Infertility	Dr Asha Baxi
International Academic Exchange	Dr Varsha Baste
MTP	Dr Bharti Maheshwari
Medical Education	Dr Abha Singh
Medical Disorders in Pregnancy	Dr Komal Chavan
Midlife Management	Dr Rajendra Nagarkatti
Oncology	Dr Bhagyalaxmi Nayak
Perinatology	Dr Vaishali Chavan
Practical Obstetrics	Dr Sanjay Das
Public Awareness	Dr Kalyan Barmade
Quiz	Dr Sebanti Goswami
Safe Motherhood	Dr N Palaniappan
Breast	Dr Sneha Bhuyar
Sexual Medicine	Dr Sudha Tandon
Urogynaecology	Dr Nita Thakre
Young Talent Promotion	Dr Vinita Singh

Contributors

Alpesh Gandhi MB DGO FRCOG FICOG
President Elect, FOGSI 2020
Senior Consultant
Obstetrics and Gynecology
Critical Care in Obstetrics Specialist
Arihant Women's Hospital
Ahmedabad, Gujarat, India

Ashwini Ingale MBBS DNB
Junior Consultant
Department of Obstetrics and Gynecology
Surya Hospitals
Mumbai, Maharashtra, India

Bharti Dhorepatil
DNB DGO FICS FICOG Dip Endoscopy(Germany)
Vice-President, FOGSI 2016
President, POGS
Chairperson, FOGSI
Consultant
Pune, Maharashtra, India

Bhaskar Pal
MBBS DGO MD DNBE MRCOG FICOG FRCOG
Chair, RCOG India East International Representative Committee
Secretary, Indian Association of Gynaecological Endoscopists
President Elect, Bengal Obstetric and Gynaecological Society
Vice-President, FOGSI 2017
Senior Consultant
Department of Obstetrics and Gynecology
Apollo Gleneagles Hospital
Kolkata, West Bengal, India

Charmila Ayyavoo
MD DGO DFP FICOG PGDCR
Director, Aditi Hospital and Parvathy Ayyavoo Fertility Centre, Trichy
Consultant, Southern Railway Hospital, Trichy
Secretary, Trichy OG Society 2012-13
Chairperson, Clinical Research Committee, FOGSI 2016-18
President, Menstrual Hygiene Management Consortium
Chennai, Tamil Nadu, India

Hrishikesh D Pai
MD FCPS FICOG MSc(USA) FRCOG
Scientific Director, Bloom IVF
Secretary General, FOGSI 2015-17
Gynecologist and Head of IVF Unit
Lilavati Hospital
Mumbai, Maharashtra, India

Jayam Kannan MD DGO FICOG
Vice-President, FOGSI 2018
Emeritus Professor
Tamil Nadu Dr MGR Medical University
Director
Garbba Rakshambigai Fertility Centre
Chennai, Tamil Nadu, India

Kamini Patel MD
Secretary, Ahmedabad Obstetrics and Gynecological Society, 2018-19
CEO
Vani IVF Centre
Ahmedabad, Gujarat, India

Kirtan M Vyas MS (Obs/Gyne)
Director
Sevak Maternity and Surgical Hospital
Ahmedabad, Gujarat, India

Mala Arora FRCOG(UK) FICOG FICMCH
Chairperson, ICOG 2017
Vice-President, FOGSI 2011
Editor-in-Chief
World Clinics in Obstetrics and Gynecology (Vol 1 to 10)
Director
NOBLE IVF Centre
Faridabad, Haryana, India

Malathi G Prasad MD MRCOG(UK)
Consultant
Department of Fetal Medicine
Trichy Fetal Medicine and Fertility Centre, Trichy
Vice-President
Trichy Obstetric and Gynecological Society, IMA, FOGSI, ATN RCOG, ISUOG
Fetal Medicine and Fertility Centre
Trichy, Tamil Nadu, India

Manisha T Kundnani MD FNB FNUS
Scientific Director
Chief Consultant and Fertility Specialist
Fertility Square
The IVF Clinic
Mumbai, Maharashtra, India

Nandita Palshetkar
MD FCPS FICOG FRCOG(UK)
President of FOGSI 2019
Scientific Director, Bloom IVF
Professor of Obstetrics and Gynecology
Dr DY Patil Medical College, Hospital
and Research Centre
Navi Mumbai, Maharashtra, India

P Prashitha MS FRM
Consultant
Garbba Rakshambigai Fertility Centre
Chennai, Tamil Nadu, India

Parzan Mistry
MS DNB FMAS MNAMS FRM FICOG
Masters in Reproductive Medicine
Clinical Associate, Bloom IVF
Consultant Obstetrician, Gynecologist and
IVF Specialist, Wockhardt Hospital,
Bhatia General Hospital, Masina Hospital
Mumbai, Maharashtra, India

Pratik Tambe MD FICOG
Chairperson
Endocrinology Committee, FOGSI 2017-19
Consultant
Mumbai, Maharashtra, India

Priya Kannan MBBS MMed MCE
President, ACE 2018-19
Embryologist
Garbba Rakshambigai Fertility Centre
Chennai, Tamil Nadu, India

Ruchi Pathak MBBS DGO FICOG
Consultant
Medical Advisor, PSIIPL
Vardaan Hospital
Varanasi, Uttar Pradesh, India

Seetha Ramamoorthy Pal
DGO MD FRCOG FICOG RCOG/RCR Diploma in
Advanced Obstetric Ultrasound
Senior Consultant
Apollo Gleneagles Hospital
Kolkata, West Bengal, India

Sejal R Naik MS(Obs/Gyne) FMAS FRM
Director
Belly and Love, Women's Care,
Athawa Gate, Surat
Consultant, Gyne-endoscopist and
Infertility Specialist
Rahul Hospital and Well Women Clinic
Surat, Gujarat, India

Sini S Venugopal MD FMAS DMAS FICMCH
ART Consultant and Endoscopic Surgeon
Managing Director and Chief Consultant
Genix Fertility Care, Bhubaneswar
Assistant Professor
HiTech Medical College and Hospital
Bhubaneswar, Odisha, India

Suchitra N Pandit
MD DNB FRCOG DFP FICOG MNAMS
President, FOGSI 2014
Senior Consultant
Department of Obstetrics and Gynecology
Surya Hospitals
Mumbai, Maharashtra, India

Sujata Misra MD(Obs/Gyne) FICOG
Vice-President, FOGSI 2015
Head
Department of Obstetrics and Gynecology
Fakir Mohan Medical College
Cuttack, Odisha, India

Sunil J Shah MD FICOG
Director
Sarvamangal Women's Hospital and
IVF Centre
Ahmedabad, Gujarat, India

Sushma S Deshmukh MD DGO
Director
Central India Test Tube Baby Centre
Deshmukh Hospital, Nagpur
Head
Department of Obstetrics and Gynecology
GetWell Multispecialty and
Research Centre
Nagpur, Maharashtra, India

Tulika Jha DGO MS(Obs/Gyne)
Associate Professor
Department of Obstetrics and Gynecology
RG Kar Medical College and Hospital
Kolkata, West Bengal, India

Foreword

'When you carry a life and it's there, and then gone, a part of your soul dies. Forever.'
—**Casey Wiegano**

The pain of loss of a child is unbearable to the parents. If there are repeated losses, the pain and agony is multi-fold. For the treating clinician, it is a difficult condition to evaluate and manage. In spite of great advances in science, the management of recurrent pregnancy loss still remains elusive. An earnest attempt has been made by the editors of this *Handbook of Recurrent Pregnancy Loss* to bring all the recent advances available for the management of this perplexing condition into this book.

Recurrent pregnancy loss may be due to many causes. Both central and local causes can contribute to this condition. This book has been structured in such a way that the reader can correlate to the different conditions and pathologies which may lead to repeated pregnancy loss. A practical approach to this condition is followed with a logical sequence which will benefit a practising physician.

'We for Stree' has been the FOGSI theme in my Presidential year, 2019. This book will serve the cause of women's health in this country as it will update the knowledge of the clinician and help to make our women 'safer, stronger and smarter' as having a living child will contribute to both her physical and emotional health.

Nandita Palshetkar MD FCPS FICOG FRCOG(UK)
President of FOGSI 2019
Scientific Director, Bloom IVF
Professor of Obstetrics and Gynecology
Dr DY Patil Medical College, Hospital and Research Centre
Navi Mumbai, Maharashtra, India

Preface

'The heart and soul of good writing is research; you should write not what you know but what you can find out about.' —**Robert J Sawyer**

This *Handbook of Recurrent Pregnancy Loss* is a unique concept and brain child of the President of FOGSI, Dr Nandita Palshetkar to bring an update on this perplexing condition. Recurrent pregnancy losses (RPL) are a distressing issue for both the couple and the clinician. There is no clarity on the definition of the condition or the investigations to be done. This condition is multifactorial and may need elaborate and extensive testing which may still not yield a cause and hence a treatment.

The chapters in this handbook have been prepared with a practical outlook. We hope it proves to be of benefit to the practising clinician and for the student. Different chapters on genetic causes, the impact of cervical factor, the effects of antiphospholipid antibodies, male factor and infections on recurrent pregnancy losses are presented and an attempt has been made to understand their contribution to this condition and the treatment options available. A separate chapter on the endocrinological perspective in recurrent pregnancy losses has been included. Investigative modalities proposed for the management of recurrent pregnancy losses such as ultrasound and hysteroscopy have also been dealt with in detail. Proposed treatment options for this condition such as progesterone therapy and heparin treatment have been discussed in this book. Newer management options which are picking up pace like preimplantation genetic diagnosis (PGD) and immunotherapy have been separately dealt with. The option of assisted conception techniques to help couples has also found mention in a separate chapter. Special chapters on setting up of an exclusive RPL clinic and tender loving care (TLC) are included as the emotional health of the sorrowing couple is equally important.

The chapters have been authored by leading clinicians and academicians from the length and breadth of the country. We are indebted to all of them for their great contribution. We hope that this handbook will spawn research and deliberations into this condition and will provide more solutions which will benefit women's health.

Jayam Kannan
Hrishikesh D Pai
Charmila Ayyavoo

Acknowledgments

Our thanks to the President of FOGSI, Dr Nandita Palshetkar, all Office Bearers of FOGSI, Co-Editors, Publishers and the sponsors of the educational grant.

Our special thanks to Dr Prateik Tambe, Chairperson, FOGSI for his untiring support and help.

Contents

1. **Definitions and Guidelines on Recurrent Pregnancy Loss** — 1
   Malathi G Prasad, Jayam Kannan

2. **Investigations in Recurrent Pregnancy Loss** — 8
   Kamini Patel, Sunil J Shah

3. **Genetic Causes of Recurrent Pregnancy Loss** — 18
   Mala Arora

4. **Role of Ultrasound in Recurrent Pregnancy Loss** — 26
   Seetha Ramamoorthy Pal

5. **Progesterones in Recurrent Pregnancy Loss** — 37
   Bharti Dhorepatil, Parzan Mistry

6. **Antiphospholipids in Recurrent Pregnancy Loss** — 45
   Bhaskar Pal, Tulika Jha

7. **Heparin in Recurrent Pregnancy Loss** — 56
   Sujata Misra, Charmila Ayyavoo

8. **Endocrinological Perspectives in Recurrent Pregnancy Loss** — 61
   Pratik Tambe, Sini S Venugopal

9. **Cervical Factors in Recurrent Pregnancy Loss** — 72
   Alpesh Gandhi, Kirtan M Vyas

10. **Hysteroscopy in Recurrent Pregnancy Loss** — 80
    Sushma S Deshmukh, Sejal R Naik

11. **Role of Male Factor in Recurrent Pregnancy Loss** — 105
    Ruchi Pathak

12. **Infections and Recurrent Pregnancy Loss** — 110
    Charmila Ayyavoo

13. **Preimplantation Genetic Diagnosis: Application and Acceptance in Recurrent Pregnancy Loss** — 118
    Priya Kannan

14. **Setting up a Recurrent Pregnancy Loss Clinic** — 124
    Suchitra N Pandit, Ashwini Ingale

15. **Role of Assisted Reproduction in Recurrent Pregnancy Loss** — 129
    Nandita Palshetkar, Manisha T Kundnani

16. **Immunotherapy in Recurrent Pregnancy Loss** — 136
    Hrishikesh D Pai, Manisha T Kundnani

17. **Tender Loving Care** — 142
    Jayam Kannan, P Prashitha

Index — 145

Chapter 1: Definitions and Guidelines on Recurrent Pregnancy Loss

Malathi G Prasad, Jayam Kannan

■ INTRODUCTION

Recurrent pregnancy loss (RPL) is not only a physical condition, it involves social, psychological, and spiritual domain of health as defined by WHO.[1] RPL is an important reproductive health issue which is physically and emotionally taxing for couples and a challenge to the treating clinicians as well. The incidence of RPL varies widely between reports because of the differences in the definitions and the criteria used as well as the population characteristics.[2] Indeed, the risk is between 9% and 12% in women aged less than 35 years but increases to 50% in women aged more than 40 years.[3] The incidence varies with the various definitions.

It is important to define recurrent miscarriage with precision as the etiology would make a large difference in evaluation, management, counseling, and prognostication of future pregnancies. Reassurance from the treating clinician is of utmost importance for the psychological wellbeing of the couple **(Table 1)**.

A prior pregnancy history is an important prognostic factor.[4] Self-reported losses may not be accurate. Successful outcome will occur in more than two-thirds of couples as in most of the cases it is unexplained.

■ DEFINITION

Primary RPL refers to multiple losses in a woman with no previous pregnancy losses beyond 20 gestational weeks whereas secondary RPL refers to multiple losses in a woman who has already had a pregnancy beyond 20 gestational weeks. Tertiary RPL refers to multiple pregnancy losses in between normal pregnancies.[5] Some clinicians do insist the definition should include RPL with the same partner.

This division is not so important as the etiological factors and prognosis is the same in two groups. Perhaps the incidence of acquired anatomical defects like uterine adhesions and cervical insufficiency may be higher in the secondary RPL group hence evaluation of the uterine cavity should be done in this group.

Most of the cases of RPL are due to more than one factor and it is termed unexplained where the cause is not identified. Early pregnancy loss, also

Table 1: Various definitions of recurrent miscarriage used in clinical trials.[6]

Reference	Definition of recurrent pregnancy loss
Cow chock 1992	2 fetal losses
Silver 1993	1 unexpected fetal death >12 weeks' gestations or 2 unexplained first trimester losses
Kutteh 1996	3 consecutive pregnancy losses
Laskin 1997	Consecutive fetal losses at <32 weeks
Rai 1997	Consecutive miscarriages
Pattison 2000	3 miscarriage
Farquharson 2002	2 fetal losses
Triolo 2003	3 consecutive fetal losses <10 weeks' gestations
Clark 2010	2 consecutive fetal losses at <24 weeks' gestation[6]

Table 2: ESHRE nomenclature of early pregnancy events.[7]

Reference	Definition of recurrent pregnancy loss
Biochemical pregnancy loss	Spontaneous pregnancy loss confirmed by decreasing beta-hCG levels but not located on ultrasound scan
Empty sac or anembryonic pregnancy loss	Intrauterine sac with absent fetal pole/yolk sac on ultrasound
Yolk sac miscarriage	Intrauterine gestational sac and yolk sac but not fetal pole on ultrasound
Embryonic miscarriage	Intrauterine gestational sac with yolk sac and fetal pole but no cardiac activity
Fetal miscarriage	Pregnancy loss >10 weeks' size with a fetal pole of CRL >33 mm on ultrasound
Ectopic pregnancy	Pregnancy visualized outside the endometrial cavity
Early pregnancy loss	Pregnancy loss <10 weeks' gestational age (<8 development weeks)
Late pregnancy loss	Greater than 12 weeks' gestation
Pregnancy of unknown location	No identifiable pregnancy on transvaginal scan with a beta-hCG level of 1,500 IU/L. No identifiable sac with on transabdominal sac with beta-hCG level of 6,000 IU/L

(CRL: crown-rump length; hCG: human chorionic gonadotropin)

referred to as miscarriage or spontaneous abortion, is defined as the loss of clinical pregnancy before 20 completed weeks of gestational age or 18 weeks after fertilization or if gestational age is unknown, the loss of an embryo/fetus of <400 g. Ectopic, molar, and biochemical pregnancies are thus not included **(Table 2)**.[3]

Preclinical Pregnancy Loss

This entity is diagnosed by performing serum beta human chorionic gonadotropin (hCG) assays in the late luteal phase prior to the onset of the next menstrual cycle.

Clinical Pregnancy Loss

Clinical pregnancy loss is defined as pregnancy loss following an ultrasound confirmation of a gestational sac.[8]
Clinical pregnancy loss is divided into:[9]
- Pre-embryonic when no fetal pole is identified (<5 weeks)
- Embryonic when a fetal pole is identified (5–10 weeks)
- Fetal >10 weeks gestation.

Miscarriage can be further classified as embryonic loss (early miscarriage) when it occurs before 10 gestational weeks and fetal loss (fetal miscarriage) when it occurs after 10 gestational weeks.[3] Mid-trimester loss occurs between 12 weeks and 28 weeks of pregnancy. The common causes are anatomical defects and antiphospholipid syndrome. These women will benefit with a hysteroscopic evaluation.[10]

Late fetal loss occurs between 28 weeks to term.[7] The most common cause is preterm labor, preterm premature rupture of membranes, preeclampsia (PE), or congenital malformations. Unexplained stillbirth is even more traumatic than unexplained RPL and merits detailed investigations to ascertain a cause. Thrombophilia screening becomes relevant in women with midtrimester and late pregnancy losses.

Recent reports of large population of women with RPL have helped to characterize the incidence and diversity of this heterogenous disorder and a definite cause of pregnancy loss can be established in over 50% of all couples after thorough evaluation.[11]

Common established causes include uterine anomalies, antiphospholipid syndrome, hormonal, metabolic disorders, and cytogenetic abnormalities. Other etiologies have been proposed but are still considered controversial such as chronic endometritis, inherited thrombophilia's, luteal phase deficiency, and high sperm DNA fragmentation levels. Over the years, evidence-based treatments such as surgical correction of uterine anomalies or aspirin and heparin for antiphospholipid syndrome[12] have improved the outcomes for couples with RPL. However almost half of the cases remain unexplained and are empirically treated using progesterone supplementation, anticoagulation, and/or immune modulatory treatments. Nowadays the invention of newer diagnostic tests like 23-chromosome microarray genetic testing of the products of conception has helped to understand the causes in most of the cases of RPL.[10]

Regardless of the cause, the long-term prognosis of couples with RPL is good and most eventually achieve a healthy live birth. However multiple pregnancy losses can have a significant psychological toll on affected couples and many efforts are being made to improve treatment and decrease the time needed to achieve a successful pregnancy.

■ GUIDELINES ON DEFINITION

RCOG (Green-top Guideline No. 17)[4,13]

Recurrent miscarriage defined as the loss of three or more consecutive pregnancies affects 1% of couples trying to conceive. It has been estimated that 1–2% of second trimester pregnancies miscarry before 24 weeks of gestation.

ESHRE Guidelines on RPL-NOV 2017[8]

A diagnosis of RPL could be considered after the loss of two or more pregnancies.

Based on evidence the evaluation may be considered either after 2 or 3 miscarriages and should be decided by the treating clinician and informed choice made by the couple. In couple with risk factors evaluation may be initiated after 2 pregnancy losses.

A pregnancy in the definition is confirmed at least by either serum or urine B-hCG, i.e. including nonvisualized pregnancy losses (biochemical pregnancy losses and/or resolved and treated pregnancies of unknown location). In the nonvisualized pregnancy loss, group pregnancy losses after gestational week 6 are included. If a pregnancy was confirmed by ultrasound and there was complete expulsion of embryo it comes under the definition of miscarriage.

Ectopic, molar pregnancies and implantation failure should not be included in the definition. Pregnancy losses both after spontaneous conception and after ART treatment should be included in the definition.

Recurrent early pregnancy loss (REPL) is the loss of two or more pregnancies before 10 weeks of gestational age.

■ TERMINOLOGY

The terminology used for pregnancy loss needs to be clear, consistent, and patient-sensitive for the purposes of this guideline. The Guideline Development Group (GDG) recommends the use of "pregnancy loss" as a general term and early embryo loss, first trimester pregnancy loss, and second trimester pregnancy loss when gestation-specific reference is needed.[2]

We recommend the use of RPL to describe repeated pregnancy demise and to reserve RPL to describe cases where all pregnancies have been confirmed as intrauterine miscarriages.

The terms spontaneous abortion, chemical pregnancy, and blighted ovum are ambiguous and should be avoided.

The use of consistent terminology and careful description of couples' reproductive history is of the utmost importance in RPL research as it is a prerequisite for comparison of studies.

The GDG concludes to use the term RPL.

BMJ Best Practice[10]

Recurrent miscarriage is defined as two or more failed clinical pregnancies (i.e. documented by ultrasound or histopathology). It affects about 1% of all fertile couples trying to conceive in comparison with sporadic nonconsecutive miscarriages which occur in about 15-20% of all pregnancies. A miscarriage includes any pregnancy that ends before the age of viability which currently stands at 24 weeks' gestation. A miscarriage that occurs before 12 weeks' gestation is commonly termed an early or first trimester miscarriage, and one that occurs between 13 weeks and 24 weeks' gestation is known as a late or second trimester miscarriage.

ASRM[14]

American Society for Reproductive Medicine defines RPL as two or more clinical pregnancy losses (documented by ultrasonography or histopathologic examination) but not necessarily consecutive.

ACOG—Up To Date[2]

The definition of RPL varies which makes studying the phenomenon and determining which couples to counsel or treat a more challenging event. As examples, varying definitions have been included:
- Two or more failed clinical pregnancies as documented by ultrasonography or histopathologic examination.
- Three consecutive pregnancy losses which are not required to be intrauterine.

The ACOG definition is clinically more relevant as most clinicians would start investigations for RPL after two consecutive losses.[9] However, this would increase the prevalence of RPL to 5% as compared to previous 1% with three or more losses. It would also favorably skew the effect of treatment modalities. Hence it is thought that for research and publication purposes, we retain the definition of three or more losses. Logically, it will be hard to retain the RCOG definition, as changing trends in clinical practice will generate data accordingly. However, this heterogenecity in definition hinders scientific research and gives birth to varying clinical practices globally. Tulandi et al. have taken up all these considerations and suggested the following, which is

acceptable in the present scenario of managing the women with pregnancy losses:[5]
- Two or more failed clinical pregnancies as documented by ultrasonography or histopathologic examination.
- Three consecutive pregnancy losses, which are not required to be intrauterine.

Recurrent implantation failure and preclinical pregnancy loss/very early pregnancy loss (VEPL) are markers of poor implantation and have a common spectrum with RPL.[10] However the current definition does not take this into consideration. This is because both these entities are in themselves not clearly defined and hence data collection can be skewed. Preclinical losses with documented beta-hCG rise and fall are a clear indication of failed implantation and may result from genetically abnormal embryos. This is the reason why some authors believe that rather than the number of losses the time of take home a baby from the time of first pregnancy event should also be taken into consideration in the definition.

Recurrent implantation failure (RIF) is defined as no implantation after transfer of 10 Grade A embryos of day 2/3 maturity or 4 blastocyst of day 5 maturity, fresh and frozen cycles included. A standard definition is still lacking.[10] This is an entity distinct from RPL although they both have many overlapping causes. They may be described as two ends of the same spectrum. Recurrent implantation failure is only relevant in the setting of assisted conception cycles whereas RPL is usually seen in spontaneous conceptions.

The incidence of acquired anatomical defects like uterine adhesions and cervical insufficiency may be higher in the secondary RPL group hence evaluation of the uterine cavity should always be done in this group.

It may also be proposed that in women greater than 37 years, one miscarriage should prompt genetic screening and replacement of a euploid embryo. Similarly, RIF, abnormal gamete morphology, poor quality embryos, and advanced maternal/paternal age should have sperm DNA fragmentation index (DFI) and preferably preimplantation genetic screening (PGS) of the trophectodermal cells and replacement of only euploid embryos prior to complete cessation of gametogenesis.

Women with a pregnancy loss will often ask "when is it best to try again?" Although the World Health Organization has recommended 6 months interpregnancy interval between pregnancies, there are studies to suggest that a shorter interpregnancy interval in women with RPL may have better outcomes.[1]

■ CONCLUSION

A thorough evaluation may be recommended after two consecutive pregnancy losses rather than three for better understanding and to ally apprehension and anxiety in the couple.

With the advent of new diagnostic strategies like 23-chromosome microarray, there is a likelihood of revision in definitions and terminologies of RPL.

With newer diagnostic tools, we are likely to evolve into newer etiologies thereby reducing the prevalence of unexplained RPL.

REFERENCES

1. World Health Organization. (2005). Report of WHO technical consultation on birth spacing. (online) Available from https://www.who.int/maternal_child_adolescent/documents/birth_spacing05/en/ [Last accessed November, 2019].
2. Kutteh WH. Recurrent pregnancy loss. Precis: An Update in Obstetrics and Gynecology. Washington DC; American College of Obstetricians and Gynecologists; 2002. pp. 151-61.
3. Stephenson MD. Frequency of factors associated with habitual abortion in 197 couples. Fertil Steril. 1996;66(1):24-9.
4. Royal College of Obstetricians and Gynaecologists. (2011). The Investigation and treatment of couples with recurrent miscarriages. Royal College of Obstetricians and Gynecologists green top guideline No. 17 May 2011. (online) Available from www.rcog.org.uk. [Last accessed November, 2019].
5. Tulandi T, Eckler K. Definition and etiology of recurrent pregnancy loss. (online) Available from https://www.uptodate.com/contents/definition-and-etiology-of-recurrent-pregnancy-loss [Last accessed November, 2019].
6. Bhattacharya S, Rajaram S, Gupta B, et al. Recurrent Miscarriage: Should the Definition be revised? Arora M, Bhattacharya S, Kumari V (Eds). World Clin Obstet Gynecol Recurrent Miscarriage. 2011;1(1).
7. Kolte AM, Bernard LA, Christiansen OB, et al. Terminology for pregnancy loss prior to viability: a consensus statement from the ESHRE early pregnancy special interest group. Hum Reprod. 2015;30(3):495-8.
8. ESHRE Early Pregnancy Guideline Development Group. (2017). ESHRE guideline on recurrent pregnancy loss.
9. Carson SA, Branch DW. Management of early recurrent pregnancy loss. ACOG Educ Bull. 2001;24:1-12.
10. Arora M, Mukhopadhaya N. Recurrent pregnancy loss. Jaypee Brothers Medical Publishers (P) Ltd. 2018 Jun 30.
11. Eastman NJ. Habitual abortion. In: Meigs JV, Sturgis SH, Taymor ML, Green TH (Eds). Progress in Gynecology, Volume 1. New York: Grune & Stratton; 1946.
12. Branch DW, Silver RM. Antiphospholipid syndrome. ACOG Educ Bull. 1998;244:302-11.
13. National Institute of Child Health and Human Development. (2012). What is pregnancy loss/miscarriage? (online) Available from https://www.nichd.nih.gov/health/topics/pregnancyloss/conditioninfo/causes [Last accessed November, 2019].
14. Practice Committee of the American society for Reproductive Medicine. Evaluation and treatment of RPL: A committee opinion. Fertil Steril. 2002;98:1103-11.

Chapter 2

Investigations in Recurrent Pregnancy Loss

Kamini Patel, Sunil J Shah

"The Bottom of your soul, you will know, is the place of your happiness"
—Miguel de Molinos

■ INTRODUCTION

Spontaneous pregnancy loss is a surprisingly common occurrence, with approximately 15% of all clinically recognized pregnancies resulting in pregnancy failure. Recurrent pregnancy loss (RPL) has been inconsistently defined. When defined as three consecutive pregnancy losses prior to 20 weeks from the last menstrual period, it affects approximately 1-2% of women **(Fig. 1)**.[1]

■ IMMUNOLOGICAL SCREENING

Human Leukocyte Antigen

Increased probability of human leukocyte antigen (HLA) compatibility was thought to produce the antibodies that protect against fetal rejection. Many studies and meta-analysis were done for allele sharing in the HLA-A, B, and C loci.

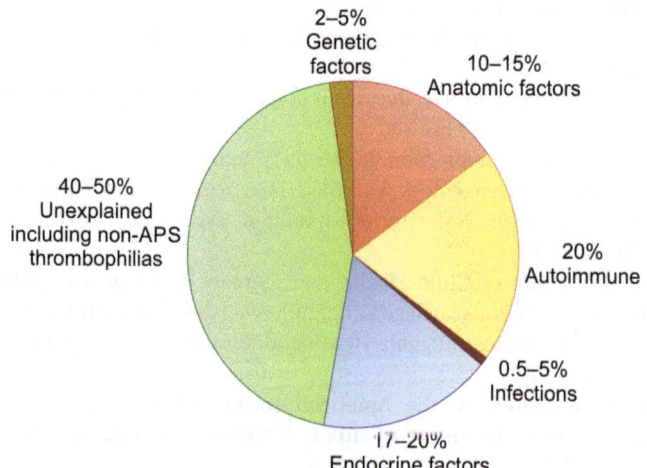

Fig. 1: Etiology of recurrent pregnancy loss.[2]

"European Society of Human Reproduction and Embryology (ESHRE)[3] recommends: HLA determination in women with RPL is not recommended in clinical practice. Only HLA class II determination could be considered in Scandinavian women with secondary RPL after the birth of a boy for prognostic purposes".

Anti-HY Antibodies

Anti-HY antibodies are antibodies directed against male-specific minor histocompatibility (HY) antigens expressed on most or all nucleated cells from males.[4]

"*ESHRE recommends*: Not to be done in clinical practice due to lack of evidences.

Cytokines

ESHRE recommends: Cytokines and cytokines polymorphism should not be used in women with RPL in clinical practices.

Antinuclear Antibodies[5]

Antinuclear antibodies (ANA) are antibodies directed against various components of the cell nuclei, often detected in patients with autoimmune diseases.

"ESHRE recommends testing for explanatory purposes as evidences found in most studies".

Natural Killer Cells

There is sufficient evidence to recommend natural killer (NK) cell testing of either peripheral blood or endometrial tissue in women with RPL.

Others Immunological Tests

- Anti-HLA antibodies
- Celiac disease serum markers
- Antisperm antibodies.

■ METABOLIC AND ENDOCRINOLOGIC FACTORS

- *Thyroid dysfunction*:
  - *Hyperthyroidism (Graves' disease)*: Some associations are noted with pregnancy losses.
  - *Hypothyroidism*: Not great association but some studies suggest association with RPL.

- *Thyroid autoantibodies*: In women with RPL, thyroid peroxidase antibodies (TPOAb) are more relevant than antibodies against the thyroid gland.

"*ESHRE recommendation*: Thyroid screening (TSH and TPO antibodies) in women with RPL. If abnormal thyroid stimulating hormone (TSH) and TPOAb levels should be followed up by T4 Testing".

- *Polycystic ovarian syndrome (PCOS) and disturbances of the insulin metabolism*: ESHRE recommends assessment of PCOS. Fasting insulin and fasting glucose assessment is not recommended.
- *Prolactin*: Some correlation noted as prolactin play role in maintaining corpus luteum and progesterone secretion.
- *Ovarian reserve testing*: Not routinely recommended.
- *Luteal phase insufficiency*: Evidences are not in favor of testing.
- *Androgens*: Not recommended.
- *Vitamin D*: One study has shown strong association but many studies did not.
- *Luteinizing hormone*: Inconsistent association so not recommended.
- *Hyperhomocysteinemia*: Due to inconsistent data and association not recommended routinely.

■ ANATOMICAL INVESTIGATION

- Anatomic abnormalities account for 10–15% of cases of RPL and are generally thought to cause miscarriage by interrupting the vasculature of the endometrium, prompting abnormal and inadequate placentation. Thus, those abnormalities that might interrupt the vascular supply of the endometrium are thought to be potential causes of RPL. These include congenital uterine anomalies, intrauterine adhesions, and uterine fibroids or polyps.[6]
- The uterine septum is the congenital uterine anomaly most closely linked to RPL, with as much as a 76% risk of spontaneous pregnancy loss among affected patients.
- *Other Müllerian anomalies*: Unicornuate, didelphic, and bicornuate uteri have been associated with smaller increases in the risk for RPL.
- The role of the arcuate uterus in causing RPL is unclear.
- The presence of intrauterine adhesions is sometimes associated with Asherman syndrome which may significantly impact placentation and result in early pregnancy loss. Intramural fibroids larger than 5 cm, as well as submucosal fibroids of any size, can cause RPL.
- Although congenital anomalies caused by prenatal exposure to diethylstilbestrol are clearly linked to RPL but this is becoming less clinically relevant as most affected patients move beyond their reproductive years.

All women with RPL should have an assessment of the uterine anatomy.

■ MALE FACTORS

Sperm quality, occupational exposure, and lifestyle such as smoking, drinking alcohol, and soft drugs should be assessed in addition to the female factors. Assessing sperm DNA fragmentation in couples with RPL can be considered for indirect evidences.

■ INFECTIOUS ETIOLOGIES

The proposed mechanisms for infectious causes of pregnancy loss include:
- Direct infection of the uterus, fetus, or placenta
- Placental insufficiency
- Chronic endometritis or endocervicitis
- Amnionitis
- Infected intrauterine device.

Those particular infections speculated to play a role in RPL include *Mycoplasma, Ureaplasma, Chlamydia trachomatis, L monocytogenes*, and *Herpes Simplex Virus 19*. The most pertinent risk for RPL secondary to infection is chronic infection in an immunocompromised patient.

Evaluation and therapy should be tailored to individual cases. If a patient with RPL has a condition that leaves her immunocompromised or a history suggestive of sexually transmitted diseases, evaluation for chronic infections may be warranted. There is no evidence that routine infectious evaluation is appropriate or productive.[7]

■ ENVIRONMENTAL ETIOLOGIES

Three particular exposures, smoking, alcohol, and caffeine, have gained particular attention, and merit special consideration given their widespread use and modifiable nature.[8]

1. *Alcohol*: Maternal alcoholism (or frequent consumption of intoxicating amounts of alcohol) is consistently associated with higher rates of spontaneous pregnancy loss while a connection with more moderate ingestion remains tenuous.
2. *Smoking*: Cigarette smoking could increase the risk of spontaneous abortion based on the ingestion of nicotine, a strong vasoconstrictor that is known to reduce uterine and placental blood flow. However, the link between smoking and pregnancy loss remains controversial, as some, but not all, studies have found an association.
3. *Caffeine*: There appears some evidence that caffeine, even in amounts as low as 3 to 5 cups of coffee per day, may increase the risk of spontaneous pregnancy loss with a dose-dependent response. The association of caffeine, alcohol, and nicotine intake with RPL is even weaker than their associations with sporadic loss.

THROMBOPHILIA

Inherited and combined inherited/acquired thrombophilias are common, with more than 15% of the white population carrying an inherited thrombophilic mutation.[9]

The most common of these are the factor V Leiden mutation, mutation in the promoter region of the prothrombin gene, and mutations in the gene encoding methylenetetrahydrofolate reductase (MTHFR).

Genetic thrombophilic factors are:
- *Factor V Leiden mutation renders factor V resistant to cleavage by activated protein C (also termed as activated protein C resistance)*: Of doubtful clinical significance.
- *Prothrombin mutation (20210GA)*: Leads to rise in plasma prothrombin concentration and thereby increases the risk of thrombosis. Some studies show significant association with prothrombin mutation and RPL.
- *Protein C, Protein S, and anti-thrombin deficiency*: Deficiency of anticoagulant protein is less common, but more strongly associated with venous thromboembolism than factor V Leiden and the prothrombin mutation.
- *Methylenetetrahydrofolate reductase (MTHFR) mutation*: No longer considered for routine assessment of thrombosis.

In contrast, more severe thrombophilic deficiencies, such as those of antithrombin and protein S, are much less common in the general population.

"ESHRE recommendation for women with RPL is not to screen for hereditary thrombophilia unless in the context of research or in women with additional risk factors for thrombophilia".

Appropriate therapy for heritable or acquired thrombophilias should be initiated once the disorder is diagnosed. Therapy is disorder-specific and includes: (1) supplemental folic acid for those patients with hyperhomocysteinemia, (2) prophylactic anticoagulation in cases of isolated defects with no personal or family history of thrombotic complications, and (3) therapeutic anticoagulation in cases of combined thrombophilic defects. Homocysteine levels should be retested after initial treatment, and prophylactic anticoagulation considered when hyperhomocysteinemia is refractory to dietary intervention.

GENETIC CAUSES (FLOWCHART 1)[10,11]

There are two common types of abnormalities that occur in early pregnancy losses: developmental and genetic abnormalities. Most pregnancies that miscarry early are morphologically abnormal. Some of these phenotypically abnormal embryos will also be genetically abnormal, as will some phenotypically normal embryos.[12]

Flowchart 1: Genetic causes.[10,11]

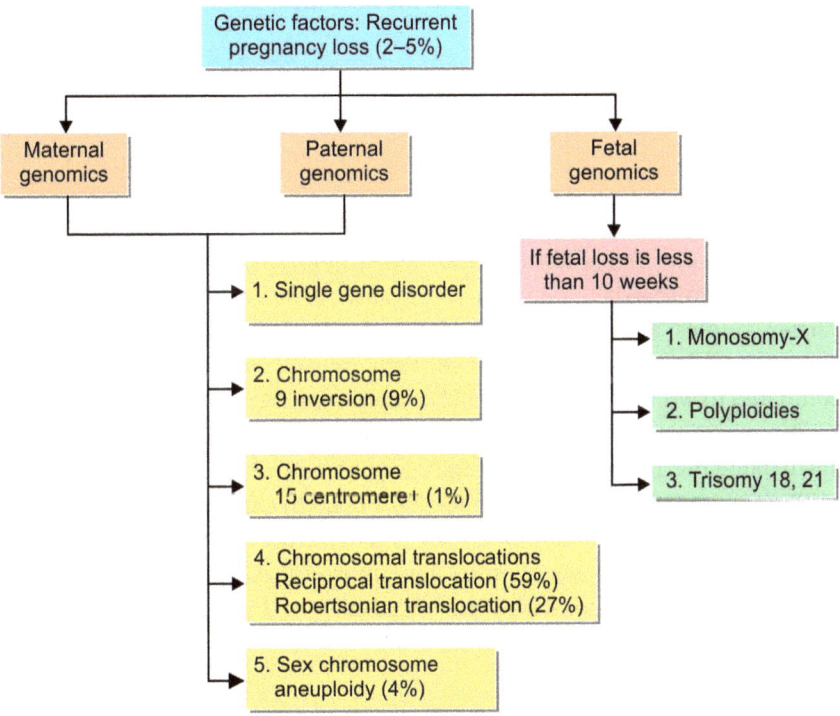

Fetal Genomics

Genetic abnormalities of the conceptus are a recognized cause of sporadic and RPL. In a systematic review, the prevalence of chromosome abnormalities in a single sporadic miscarriage was 45% (95% CI 38–52; 13 studies; 7012 samples).[13]

It is possible to ascertain whether an early pregnancy loss is due to a genetically abnormal embryo or fetus (aneuploidy) by analyzing the pregnancy or fetal tissue.[14] Published studies have used a variety of genetic techniques [conventional karyotyping, fluorescence in situ hybridization (FISH), or array-based comparative genomic hybridization (array-CGH)]. Analysis by conventional karyotyping is limited by the failure of tissue culture and the fact that it does not distinguish between maternal contamination and a normal (euploid) female fetus.[15] FISH is limited as it only uses probes for certain chromosomes, and therefore does not necessarily detect the chromosomal cause of the miscarriage. Array comparative genomic hybridization (CGH) is a better technique, and currently preferred technique, looking at all chromosomes and avoiding the limitations associated with karyotype and FISH.[14] New techniques such as next generation sequencing

(NGS) have not yet been extensively investigated in genetic analysis of pregnancy tissue but may be useful in the near future.[16]

Parental Genetic Analysis

Abnormal parental karyotypes were found in around 1.9% of couples (n = 20432) referred for genetic testing after recurrent pregnancy loss in a large retrospective cohort study.[17,18]

In another retrospective study of 795 couples with two or more pregnancy losses, chromosomal abnormalities were found in 3.5% of the couples. The subsequent miscarriage rate was higher and the live birth rate was lower in carrier couples, although the cumulative live birth rate was 64%.[19] Another cohort study reported a lower live birth rate in carrier couples (63.0%) compared to women with a normal karyotype (78.7%).

A proportion (15.1%/17.8%) of carrier couples opts not to try to conceive again following an abnormal parental karyotype result.[17,19]

In noncarriers, the proportion was only 6%.[17] In carrier couples, the main reasons to not try to conceive were the risk of having a child with congenital abnormalities and not wanting to have more miscarriages, in noncarrier couples, the main reasons were advanced maternal age and fear of further miscarriages.[17]

Unexplained RPL

Fifty percent of the recurrent miscarriage is usually idiopathic and the possible etiologies that may be responsible for such cases may include fetal chromosome anomalies, endometrial receptivity, and genetic factors. Repetitive fetal anomalies due to increasing maternal age may result in a miscarriage, while abnormal morphological development of the endometrium in the luteal phase has been pointed out to be the cause in some of the studies.

Investigations

- Primary investigations would be karyotyping of the parents.
- Preimplantation genetic diagnosis (PGD)/preimplantation genetic screening (PGS) would be an option in case of the fetal chromosome anomalies.
- Testing of inherited thrombophilias—like factor V Leiden, prothrombin gene mutation, activated protein creatinine, homocysteine, protein C, protein S, and antithrombin III are optional and often very expensive.
- Full genome analysis done by NGS of the parents and the embryos can help in finding the unknown causes of the RPL, in knowing the single

nucleotide polymorphisms and other point mutations leading to the pregnancy loss. This test is also expensive.
- NGS with developing technologies might be easily available at lower cost as it is it the need of the hour due to increasing awareness regarding the underlying genetic causes in such cases.

Management

- Couples with chromosomal abnormalities should be referred to a clinical geneticist with whom the options of prenatal diagnosis, PGD, donor gametes, and adoption in subsequent pregnancies should be discussed.
- The probability of a successful pregnancy and the risk of a chromosomally abnormal but viable fetus vary with specific chromosomes involved and the location of the translocated segments.
- The karyotyping of the affected partner allows the prediction of the most likely segregation pattern for a specific translocation and estimate the risk of the unbalanced offspring.

■ CONCLUSION

- Spontaneous pregnancy loss is common, with approximately 15% of all clinically recognized pregnancies resulting in miscarriage.
- When RPL is defined as three consecutive pregnancy losses prior to 20 weeks from the last menstrual period, 1-2% of women will be affected.
- Because the risk of subsequent miscarriages is similar among women that have had 2 versus 3 miscarriages, and the probability of finding a treatable etiology is similar among the two groups, most experts agree that there is a role for evaluation after two losses.
- Accepted etiologies for RPL include parental chromosomal abnormalities, untreated hypothyroidism, uncontrolled diabetes mellitus, certain uterine anatomic abnormalities, and the antiphospholipid antibody syndrome (APS). Other probable or possible etiologies include additional endocrine disorders, heritable and/or acquired thrombophilias, immunologic abnormalities, and environmental causes. After evaluation for these causes, more than 33% of all cases will remain unexplained.
- Diagnostic evaluation should include maternal and paternal karyotypes, assessment of the uterine anatomy, and evaluation for thyroid dysfunction, APS, and selected thrombophilias. In some women, evaluation for insulin resistance, ovarian reserve, antithyroid antibodies, and prolactin disorders may be indicated.
- Therapy should be directed toward any treatable etiology, and may include IVF with PGD, use of donor gametes, surgical correction of anatomic

abnormalities, correction of endocrine disorders, and anticoagulation or folic acid supplementation.
- In cases of unexplained RPL, progesterone has been shown to be beneficial in decreasing the miscarriage rate in women who had experienced at least three losses. Low-dose aspirin benefits those with a history of losses at more than 13 weeks of gestation.
- Antenatal counseling and psychological support should be offered to all couples experiencing RPL, as these measures have been shown to increase pregnancy success rates.
- Prognosis will depend on the underlying cause for pregnancy loss and the number of prior losses. Patients and physicians can be encouraged by the overall good prognosis, as even after four consecutive losses a patient has a greater than 60–65% chance of carrying her next pregnancy to term.

■ REFERENCES

1. El Hachem H, Crepaux V, May-Panloup P, et al. Recurrent pregnancy loss: current perspectives. Int J Women's Health. 2017;9:331-45.
2. Ford HB, Schust DJ. Recurrent pregnancy loss: etiology, diagnosis, and therapy. Rev Obstet Gynecol. 2009;2(2):76-83.
3. The ESHRE Guideline Group on RPL; Atik RB, Christiansen OB, Elson J, et al. ESHRE guideline: recurrent pregnancy loss. Hum Reprod Open. 2018;2018(2).
4. Fox-Lee L, Schust DJ. Recurrent pregnancy loss. In: Berek JS (Ed). Berek and Novak's Gynaecology. Philadelphia: Lippincott Williams and Wilkins; 2007. pp. 1277-322.
5. Miyakis S, Lockshin M, Atsumi T, et al. International consensus statement on an update of the classification criteria for definite antiphospholipid syndrome (APS). J Thromb Haemost. 2006;4(2):295-306.
6. Lin P. Reproductive outcomes in women with uterine anomalies. J Women's Health. 2004;13(1):33-9.
7. Summers P. Microbiology relevant to recurrent miscarriage. Clin Obstet Gynecol. 1994;37(3):722-9.
8. Rasch V. Cigarette, alcohol, and caffeine consumption: risk factors for spontaneous abortion. Acta Obstetricia Et Gynecologica Scandinavica. 2003;82(2):182-8.
9. Greer I. Thrombophilia: implications for pregnancy outcome. Thromb Res. 2003;109(2-3):73-81.
10. Hyde K, Schust D. Genetic considerations in recurrent pregnancy loss. Cold Spring Harb Perspect Med. 2015;5(3):a023119.
11. Page J, Silver R. Genetic causes of recurrent pregnancy loss. Clin Obstet Gynecol. 2016;59(3):498-508.
12. Warren J, Silver R. Genetics of pregnancy loss. Clin Obstet Gynecol. 2008;51(1):84-95.
13. van den Berg M, van Maarle M, van Wely M, et al. Genetics of early miscarriage. Biochim Biophys Acta Mol Basis Dis. 2012;1822(12):1951-9.

14. Mathur N, Triplett L, Stephenson M. Miscarriage chromosome testing: utility of comparative genomic hybridization with reflex microsatellite analysis in preserved miscarriage tissue. Fertil Steril. 2014;101(5):1349-52.
15. Robberecht C, Schuddinck V, Fryns J, et al. Diagnosis of miscarriages by molecular karyotyping: benefits and pitfalls. Genet Med. 2009;11(9): 646-54.
16. Shamseldin H, Swaid A, Alkuraya F. Lifting the lid on unborn lethal Mendelian phenotypes through exome sequencing. Genet Med. 2012;15(4): 307-9.
17. Franssen M, Korevaar J, van der Veen F, et al. Reproductive outcome after chromosome analysis in couples with two or more miscarriages: case-control study. BMJ. 2006;332(7544):759-63.
18. Barber J, Cockwell A, Grant E, et al. Is karyotyping couples experiencing recurrent miscarriage worth the cost?. BJOG: An International Journal of Obstetrics & Gynaecology. 2010;117(7):885-8.
19. Flynn H, Yan J, Saravelos S, et al. Comparison of reproductive outcome, including the pattern of loss, between couples with chromosomal abnormalities and those with unexplained repeated miscarriages. J Obstet Gynaecol Res. 2013;40(1):109-16.

Chapter 3: Genetic Causes of Recurrent Pregnancy Loss

Mala Arora

■ INTRODUCTION

Recurrent pregnancy loss (RPL) is a multifactorial disorder with identifiable causes in over 60% of cases. A battery of tests is recommended to rule out the various causes listed in **Table 1**.

Genetic causes were earlier thought to contribute in a small percentage, however they are assuming greater importance and it is believed that a large percentage of hitherto unexplained causes of RPL show subtle genetic abnormalities in the embryo **(Figs. 1 and 2)**. *To date, genetic evaluation of the products of conception (POC) remains the most neglected yet vital investigation.*

Table 1: Causes of recurrent miscarriage.

Lifestyle factors	• Maternal age > 35 years • Maternal obesity BMI > 30 • Paternal age
Immunological—autoimmune	• Primary antiphospholipid syndrome • Secondary antiphospholipid syndrome—systemic lupus erythematosus, autoimmune thyroiditis
Immunological—alloimmune (classified as unexplained)	• Abnormalities of cytokine production—lack of shift of Th1 to Th2 response • Lack of alpha V beta 3 integrin • Increased levels of tumor necrosis factor (TNF) alpha in the endometrium • Increased uterine natural killer cells • Sharing of human leukocyte antigens
Genetic	• Fetal trisomy, polyploidy, monosomy • Parental balanced translocations, inversions, deletions, duplications • Skewed inactivation of X chromosome • Single gene defects, e.g. alpha thalassemia major, Rett syndrome, etc.

Contd...

Contd...

Hormonal	• Polycystic ovarian syndrome • Luteal phase defects • Hyperandrogenism • Hypothyroidism/hyperthyroidism • Hyperprolactinemia • Low anti-müllerian hormone/poor ovarian reserve • Adrenal hyperplasia/Addison's disease • Deficiency of vitamin D • Uncontrolled diabetes mellitus
Anatomical	• Müllerian abnormalities, septate uterus • Fibroids—submucous, intramural • Uterine synechiae and polyps • T-shaped uterus • Cervical incompetence
Inherited thrombophilia	• Antithrombin III deficiency • Deficiency of protein C and protein S • Activated protein C resistance • Factor V Leiden mutation • Methyl tetrahydrofolate gene homozygosity and hyperhomocysteinemia • Prothrombin gene mutation • Plasminogen activator inhibitor
Semen factors	• High sperm DNA fragmentation index • Y chromosomal microdeletions
Infections	• Genital bacterial vaginosis, tuberculosis • Male urogenital infections • Systemic syphilis, Lyme's disease, toxoplasmosis, brucellosis
Systemic conditions	• Hypertension • Chronic renal disease • Chronic pulmonary disease • Heart disease • Severe rhesus sensitization
Miscellaneous	• Smoking, alcohol, drugs • Exposure to irradiation • Exposure to environmental toxins, pesticides, DDT, dry cleaning chemicals • Exposure to anesthetic gases • Environmental endocrine disrupters
Idiopathic	• Epigenetic modifications of the embryo • Maternal stress

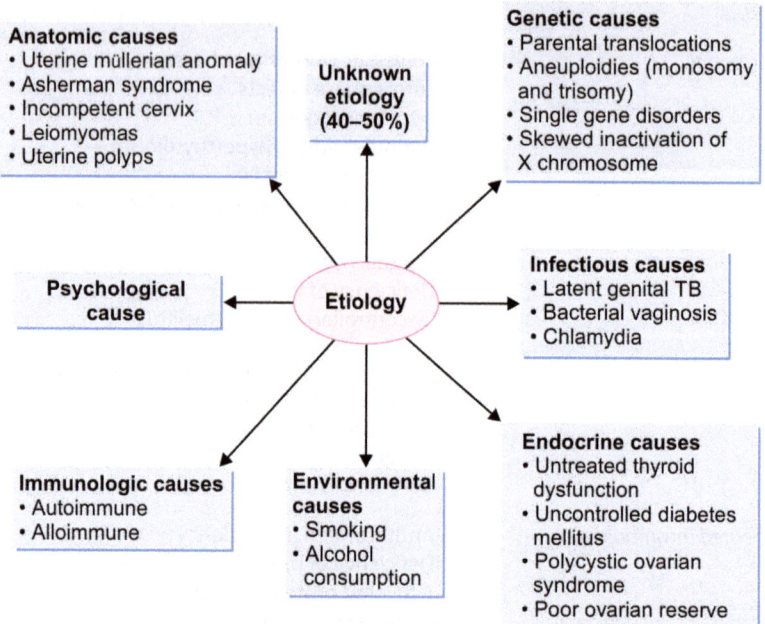

Fig. 1: Etiology of recurrent miscarriages.
Source: Ford HB, Schust DJ. Recurrent pregnancy loss: etiology, diagnosis, and therapy. Reviews in obstetrics and gynecology. 2009;2(2):76.

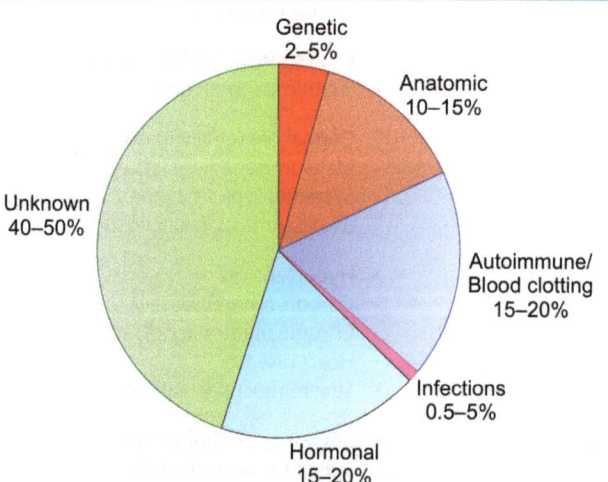

Fig. 2: Percentage-wise distribution of etiology of recurrent miscarriages.

■ TIMING OF MISCARRIAGE

The hallmark of genetic miscarriages is that they occur early between 5 weeks and 7 weeks of pregnancy. Often they may present as chemical pregnancies, empty gestational sac/anembryonic pregnancy which makes genetic evaluation of the fetus impossible.

SOURCE OF GENETIC ABNORMALITIES

There are two distinct sources of genetic abnormalities:
- Those that develop *de novo* during embryogenesis. They result from breakage of spindle fibers during mitosis leading to chromosomal aneuploidies. They are not recurrent and are by far more common of the two. They carry a good prognosis for future pregnancy outcome.
- Those associated with a *balanced translocation* in one of the parents. The parents are often carriers of balanced translocation that gets unbalanced during gametogenesis. This causes recurrent abnormal embryo formation hence the prognosis is poorer.

Prevalence of genetic abnormalities in sporadic miscarriages is estimated to be 45% (CI 38-52%) and in recurrent miscarriages 39% (CI 29-50%) in a systematic review.[1]

MODALITIES OF GENETIC TESTS

The modalities that are currently available include:
- *Fluorescent in situ hybridization (FISH)*: This can be performed in nonviable chorionic tissue. Although classically employed to detect aneuploidies of five chromosomes, i.e. 21, 18, 13, X, and Y. It can be extended to include other chromosomes, e.g. 16 and 22, which are important causes of pregnancy loss. Since it can only detect chromosomal number variations, hence may miss other genetic abnormalities.
- *Conventional karyotyping*: This requires viable chorionic tissue and hence cannot be applied to missed miscarriages. It is expensive and on many occasions the culture of chorionic tissue may fail. Another major disadvantage is that it is unable to distinguish between maternal cell contamination and fetal tissue, thereby generating a normal female karyotype report if maternal tissue contamination is heavy.
- *Microarray*-based tests include *comparative genomic hybridization (CGH)* and *single nucleotide polymorphism (SNP)* microarray. These are currently recommended as they can detect 4.4-10% additional chromosomal rearrangements compared to karyotyping. It studies all 24 chromosomes, does not require viable tissue, and can even distinguish maternal cell contamination. It can further be expanded to study single gene disorders when combined with SNP array. According to a recent publication, adding this test to the list of mandatory tests will establish a cause in 90% of miscarriages as opposed to 50%.[2] This is also used to detect certain genes expressed only in the placenta, and are implicated in RPL. Limitation of this technique is that it may not detect balanced translocations and low level of mosaicism.[3]

- *Next-generation sequencing (NGS):*[4] This is the most advanced technique, which can check till a resolution of a single base pair. It does not require viable chorionic tissue. It has the highest sensitivity to detect mosaicism. In a recent study, embryos reported as euploid by other tests were tested by NGS and 31.6% were found to be mosaic.[5]
- *Parental karyotyping*: This is not routinely recommended for all couples with RPL, as the incidence of finding an abnormal karyotype is only 1.9%. It is definitely indicated in couples with two or more pregnancy losses where genetic abnormality is detected on POC, previous offspring with a genetic abnormality, or a family history of a genetically abnormal child.[6] It is currently recommended to study not only the maternal and paternal genome but also the placental genome in RPL.

■ RECOMMENDATION

Genetic testing is still not recommended for the first pregnancy loss as this could be a sporadic loss. It is beneficial to screen the second and subsequent losses. It is now recommended to screen not only the index pregnancy but also any tissue saved from previous losses as paraffin blocks.

■ ADVANTAGES OF GENETIC TESTING

Performing genetic tests has the following advantages:
- It provides the couple with a reason for miscarriage, hence alleviates their grief.
- It can open the options of assisted reproduction with preimplantation genetic screening (PGS) in couples with balanced translocations and/or recurrent aneuploid losses.
- In couples with balanced translocation in parents and recurrent aneuploid embryos, it justifies the use of donor gametes.
- If miscarriage occurs inspite of specific treatment of an identifiable cause, genetic testing of POC will provide an explanation for failure of treatment if the products of conception show a genetic abnormality.
- It prognosticates couples with RPL. If there are recurrent euploid miscarriages, one needs to focus on identifying auterotonic cause. These couples often have a worse prognosis than those with recurrent aneuploid miscarriages.

■ TREATMENT OPTIONS

- *Genetic counseling* should be offered to all couples where a genetic abnormality is identified in the fetus. This includes a detailed family history, drawing up a pedigree, and estimating a risk of recurrence of the genetic disorder.

- *Assisted reproduction*: In couples that are carriers of balanced translocation that require donor gametes the option of intrauterine insemination (IUI) and/or in vitro fertilization (IVF) should be considered. Other indications for ART in RPL are outlined in **Table 2**.
- *Preimplantation genetic diagnosis (PGD)* is performed for couples with known carrier state of single gene disorders, there is a definite role of IVF with targeted PGD and replacement of only normal embryos, e.g. hemophilia.
- *Preimplantation genetic screening* is performed for couples with RPL. Embryo biopsy is performed post-IVF cycle to screen for aneuploidy. This has been recommended as a treatment option for couples with recurrent aneuploid miscarriages. Blastomere biopsy on day 3 (8-cell embryos) and FISH analysis was earlier employed. However, with the advent of blastocyst culture, biopsy from the trophectoderm (TE) is less traumatic and performing array CGH offers more comprehensive screening.

Blastomere biopsy yielded lower pregnancy rates whereas TE biopsy does not seem to reduce the clinical pregnancy rate. A recent study evaluated PGS versus expectant management (EM) in couples with RPL and found that live birth rate is lower and clinical miscarriage rate is higher in the EM group suggesting that PGS reduces clinical miscarriage. Murugappan et al.[7] concluded that those couples that cancelled their PGS had a higher clinical miscarriage rate than those that underwent PGS.

The argument against PGS is that many embryos in the early stage may show mosaicism. Transfer of mosaic embryos has resulted in live births with

Table 2: Indications for ART in RPL.

Indication	Procedure
Mother diagnosed to be a balanced translocation carrier	IVF donor oocytes
Advanced maternal age	IVF donor oocytes
Premature ovarian failure	IVF donor oocytes
Patients requiring PGS/PGD	IVF/autologous gametes/PGD
Male factors requiring ICSI like reduced capacitation Reduced fertilization potential	ICSI
In correctable uterine factors	Surrogacy
Recurrent implantation failure	Blastocyst culture Assisted hatching
Immunological	IVF multiple embryo replacement

(ART: assisted reproductive technology; ICSI: intracytoplasmic sperm injection; IVF: in vitro fertilization; PGS: preimplantation genetic screening; PGD: preimplantation genetic diagnosis; RPL: recurrent pregnancy loss)

Flowchart 1: Workup for early recurrent pregnancy loss.[9]

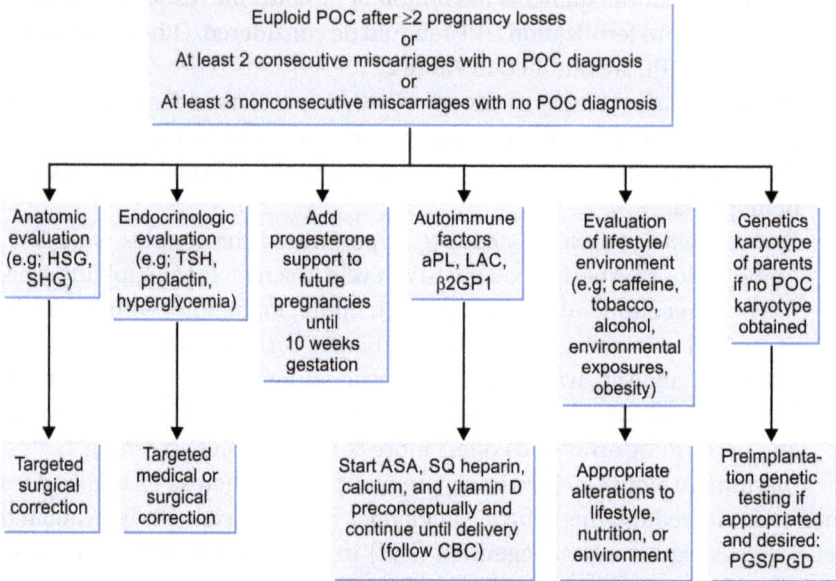

(aPL: antiphospholipid; ASA: aspirin; HSG: hysterosalpingogram; LAC: lupus anticoagulant; PGS: preimplantation genetic screening; PGD: preimplantation genetic diagnosis; POC: products of conception; SHG: sonohysterogram; TSH: thyroid-stimulating hormone)
Source: Kutteh WM, Brezina P. Recurrent pregnancy loss. Clin Reprod Med Surg; 2013. pp. 197-208.

normal offspring. Hence, in a meta-analysis it is concluded that degree of TE mosaicism was a poor predictor of ongoing pregnancy and miscarriage.[8]

■ CONCLUSION

Further good quality trials are required to clarify the indications and limitations of PGS.

Flowchart 1 outlines the investigations and treatment options in a patient with RPL.

■ REFERENCES

1. Van den Berg MM, van Maarle MC, van Wely M, et al. Genetics of early miscarriage. Biochim Biophys Acta. 2012;1822:1951-9.
2. Khalife D, Ghazeeri G, Kutteh W. Review of current guidelines for recurrent pregnancy loss: new strategies for optimal evaluation of women who may be superfertile. Semin Perinatol. 2019;43(2).105-15.
3. Sahoo T, Dzidic N, Strecker MN, et al. Comprehensive genetic analysis of pregnancy loss by chromosomal microarrays: outcomes, benefits, and challenges. Genet Med. 2017;19:83-9.

4. Shamseldin HE, Swaid A, Alkuraya FS. Lifting the lid on unborn lethal Mendelian phenotypes through exome sequencing. Genet Med. 2013;15:307-9.
5. Maxwell SM, Colls P, Hodes-Wertz B, et al. Why do euploid embryos miscarry? A case controlled study comparing the rate of miscarriage or live birth using next generation sequencing. Fertil Steril. 2016;106(6):1414-9e5.
6. Franssen MT, Korevaar JC, Leschot NJ, et al. Selective chromosome analysis in couples with two or more miscarriages: case control study. BMJ. 2005;331: 137-41.
7. Murugappan G, Shahine LK, Perfetto CO, et al. Intent to treat analysis of in vitro fertilisation and preimplantation genetic screening versus expectant management in patients with recurrent pregnancy loss. Hum Reprod. 2016;31(8):1688-74.
8. Kushnir V, Darmon S, Barad D, et al. Degree of mosaicism in trophectoderm does not predict pregnancy potential: A corrected analysis of pregnancy outcomes following transfer of mosaic embryos. Reprod Biol Endocrinol. 2018;16(1):6.
9. Kutteh WM, Brezina P. Recurrent pregnancy loss. Clin Reprod Med Surg. 2013. pp. 197-208.

Chapter 4

Role of Ultrasound in Recurrent Pregnancy Loss

Seetha Ramamoorthy Pal

■ INTRODUCTION

Recurrent pregnancy loss (RPL) includes all pregnancy losses (PLs) from the time of conception until 24 weeks of gestation. It is a very distressing and disturbing problem both for the couple and treating physician and very often there is no cause found in about 50% of the couples and no obvious solutions. Although investigations are ideally recommended after two spontaneous losses, the decision on when to start investigations will have to be decided by the doctor and the couple, as the result of shared decision-making, and be compliant with available resources.

Ultrasound is and remains the cornerstone of evaluation in RPL. It is done either as part of the investigation protocol or once pregnancy test is positive, to confirm detection of the sac and viability. One of the etiological factors that are particularly rewarding to diagnose and treat is the anatomic abnormalities of the uterus. An abnormal uterine structure is the most common cause in second trimester pregnancy losses and second most cause in first trimester losses. Acquired and congenital uterine abnormalities account for 10–15% of RPL. Depending on the type of abnormality, there are associations with cervical incompetence, preterm birth, breech presentation and growth restriction to varying degrees.[1]

Ultrasound can be helpful in different ways:
- Two-dimensional (2D) transvaginal pelvic ultrasound
- Saline infusion sonohysterography
- Three-dimensional ultrasound.

■ TRANSVAGINAL ULTRASOUND

It forms the basic first-line investigation in cases of RPL. It helps in assessing the structure of the uterus and to detect any fibroids if present. Most fibroids are not the cause of RPL. However transvaginal ultrasound is very useful in evaluating the size, site, number, and vascularity of fibroids.

It is also useful in detecting intrauterine polyps and endometrial irregularities that might suggest adhesions. It presents a sensitivity of 100% and specificity of 80% when studying uterine anomalies.[2] The markers for uterine anomaly in conventional ultrasound include a double endometrial echo complex, a wide transverse uterine diameter, and rarely a distinctive uterine duality.[3] 3D ultrasound can be further used for suspected cases of uterine anomalies, better delineation of fibroids, and accurate detection of polyps, if necessary.

Transvaginal ultrasound helps in assessing the cervical length and is considered the gold standard by the American Congress of Obstetrics and Gynaecology, the Society for Maternal and Fetal Medicine, and Society of Obstetricians and Gynaecologists of Canada. It can also help in evaluating the ovaries and adnexa.

It is important to note here that assessment of polycystic ovarian syndrome is not recommended in women with RPL to improve next pregnancy outcome.

However, women with a history of second-trimester pregnancy losses and suspected cervical weakness should be offered serial cervical sonographic surveillance.[4] Cervical length assessment is performed between 14 weeks and 24 weeks of gestation. If the cervical length is <25 mm before 24 weeks, then cerclage or progesterone is offered **(Figs. 1 A and B)**.

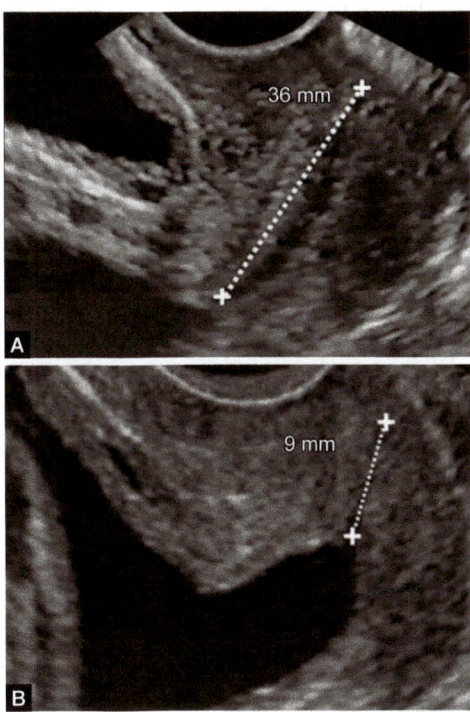

Figs. 1A and B: Normal/short cervix (Fetal Medicine Foundation).
Source: Fernandez M, House M, Jambawalikar S, et al. Investigating the mechanical function of the cervix during pregnancy using finite element models derived from high-resolution 3D MRI. Comput Methods Biomech Biomed Engin. 2016;19(4):404-17.

■ HYSTEROSONOGRAPHY

It consists of the introduction of a water-soluble contrast (physiological saline) into the cavity, so when the contrast distends the cavity, any anomaly can be seen. The advantage of the sonolucent fluid is that it better delineates hyperechogenic surface of the endometrium.[5] This is combined with 2D to detect problems. The first observation is made of the uterine cavity and the catheter placement is confirmed. In this stage, one can observe the morphology of the uterus and endometrial lining. Representative images of the uterus in sagittal and transverse planes help in detection of duplication anomalies. This however fails to differentiate septate from bicornuate uterus. Combined with 3D ultrasound, it enables better assessment of the uterine cavity. Similarly, color or power Doppler ultrasound can be used for visualization of the shape of the uterine cavity. Following distention of the uterine cavity, 2D and 3D ultrasound are used to detect focal intracavitary lesions such as endometrial polyp or submucous fibroid **(Figs. 2A and B)**.[5] Bands of fibrous tissue bridging the uterine cavity, intrauterine adhesions are usually not seen on a native ultrasound but become visible following enhancement with contrast medium.

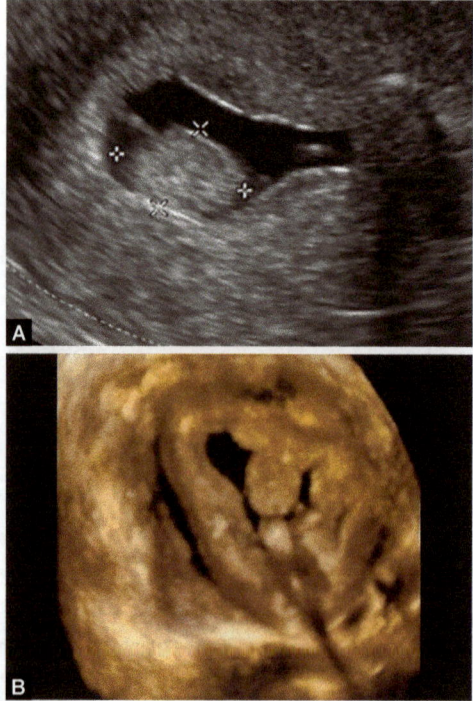

Figs. 2A and B: Hysterosonography showing endometrial polyp.

■ THREE-DIMENSIONAL ULTRASOUND

All women with RPL should have an assessment of the uterine anatomy.[4] The preferred and gold standard technique to evaluate the uterus is transvaginal 3D ultrasound, which has a high sensitivity and specificity (100%).

The first publications in regards to the potential of 3D of confirming the internal structure of the uterus, as seen by means of hysterosalpingography (HSG), date back to 1995.[6] In one of the early pioneering studies, Campbell et al. found agreement between 3D ultrasound and HSG in all cases, and moreover, considered that 3D ultrasound further aided the differential diagnosis between the subseptated and bicornuate uteri, because of the ability to assess the external contour.

When compared with 3D, 2D ultrasound is a sensitive method for diagnosing Müllerian malformations, but it cannot really differentiate between the various subtypes as it provides limited view of the uterine fundus. HSG provides information of the contour of the uterine cavity and tubal pathology, but it lacks specificity in detailing lateral fusion anomalies, and also it involves radiation.[7]

Three-dimensional transvaginal ultrasound has become nowadays the method of choice in assessing the uterus, due to many reasons and having distinct advantages over all other techniques:

- It allows the visualization of the coronal plane of the uterus, which is critical in the diagnosis of uterine anomalies, and impossible to achieve in 2D ultrasound.[8,9] The coronal view enables the clinician to examine both the endometrial cavity and uterine fundus, thus providing a complete assessment of uterine morphology **(Figs. 3A and B)**.[10-14]
- It is noninvasive, accurate, and reliable with no ionizing radiation.
- It provides exceptionally clear high resolution frontal view of the uterus and its anatomical details, including details on the uterine walls, the assessment of the relationship between endometrium and myometrium of the uterine fundus and depicts cornual angles.
- Ir provides accurate simultaneous assessment of both internal and external contour of the uterus.
- It has no side effects, so it is repeatable and is cost-effective.
- It is simple with a short and abrupt learning curve, due to higher resolution and convenience of the systems used in daily practice.
- It carries no anesthetic or surgical risks.
- It has a continuously wider availability worldwide.
- It allows storage of volume data (useful in retrospective analysis, network consultation and exchange of the data, interactive review at any time without presence of the patient, reduction of the imaging time).
- It has the characteristic of multiplanar capability, rotation and magnification, enabling an unlimited number of scan planes for detailed exploration of the uterine cavity.
- It delineates the entire cervical canal.

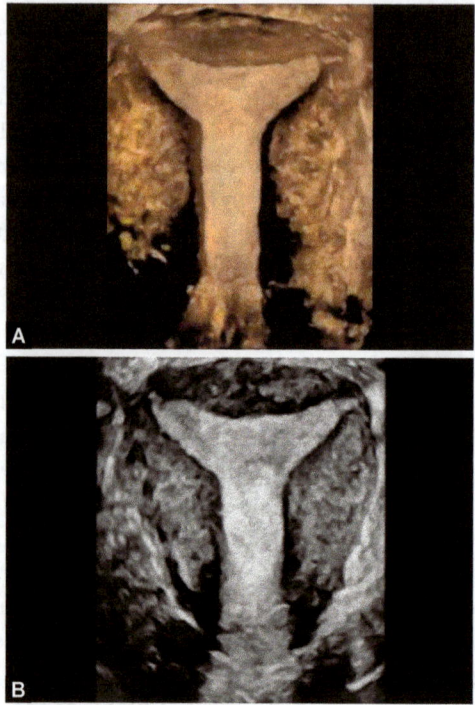

Figs. 3A and B: Three-dimensional image of normal uterus.

Three-dimensional transvaginal ultrasound has very few disadvantages: it is operator-dependent, needs expertise, and not useful in the rare situation of complete transversal vaginal septa.

Congenital anomalies of the uterus result from failure in either the organogenesis phase, fusion phase or septal resorption phase of the development of the paramesonephric or Müllerian ducts. A review of large number of studies concluded that congenital uterine anomaly was present in 4.3% (range from 2.7% to 16.7%) of the general population of fertile women and in 12.6% (range from 1.8% to 37.6%) of patients with RPL as the primary cause.[15] Various classification systems have been proposed in the field of congenital uterine anomalies. The American Fertility Society (AFS) (1998), based on the previous work of Buttram and Gibbons (1979), classified the anomalies of the female reproductive tract into groups according to the degree of failure of normal development with possible prognoses for their reproductive performance.[16] Further, Troiano and his team published a new 3D-US based method, with the purpose to help this delineation in 2004. However this has not been clinically validated yet **(Figs. 4A to C)**.[17]

The most recent classification is the ESHRE/ESGE which is based on anatomy and more clinically oriented **(Fig. 5)**.[18]

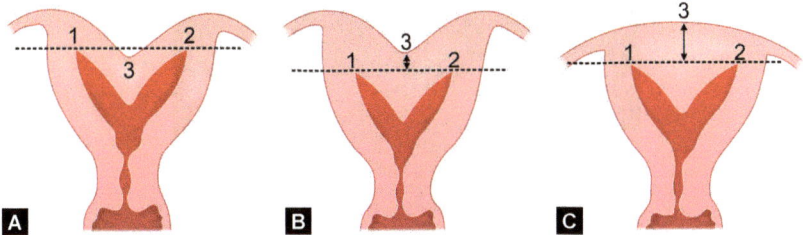

Figs. 4A to C: Classification criteria for ultrasound differentiation of septate from bicornuate uteri.[17]

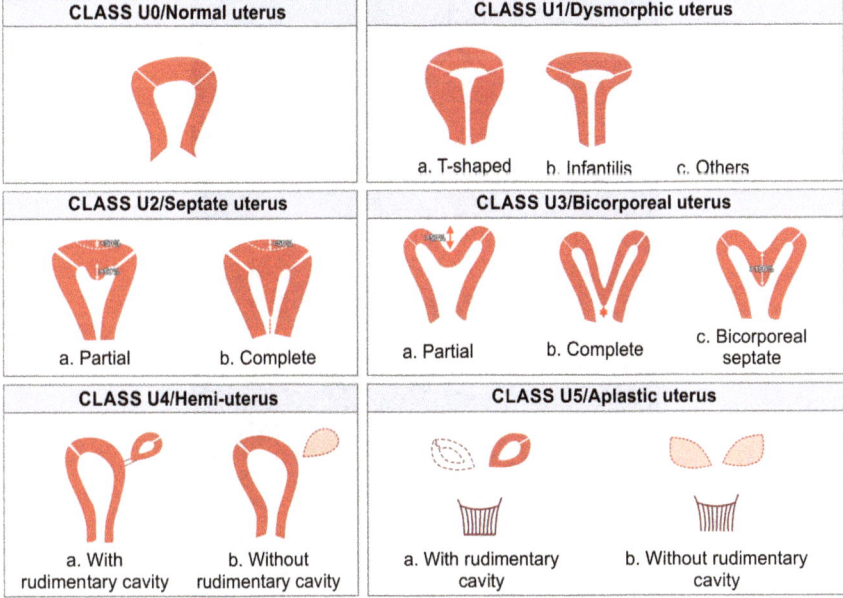

Fig. 5: ESHRE/ESGE classification of uterine anomalies. Schematic representation (Class U2: internal indentation >50% of the uterine wall thickness and external contour straight or with indentation <50%, Class U3: external indentation >50% of the uterine wall thickness, Class U3b: width of the fundal indentation at the midline >150% of the uterine wall thickness).

Among the various anomalies, septate uterus is the most common uterine anomaly associated with RPL and is associated with the poorest reproductive outcome, with a miscarriage rate of 45–60%, if left untreated. The next common anomaly associated with RPL is the bicornuate uterus which contributes to around 36% cases of RPL, followed by arcuate uterus (25%).[19]

To obtain a proper 3D image, the examination is first done with 2D ultrasound with a midsagittal cut, adjusting the capturing window so that an optimal 3D volume is obtained **(Figs. 6A to D)**.[19] This region of interest

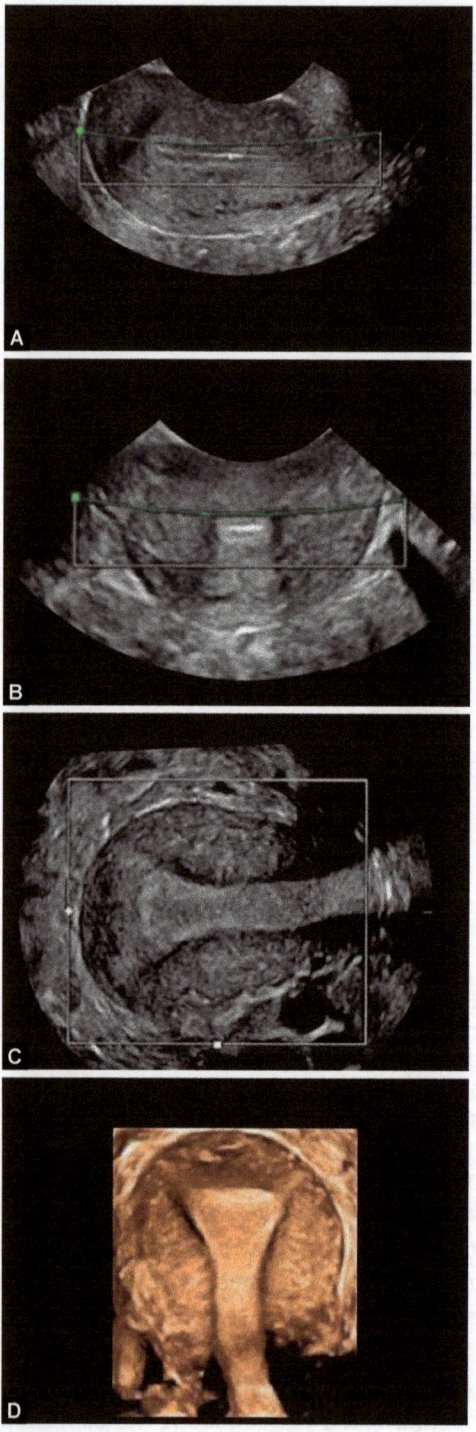

Figs. 6A to D: Obtaining a three-dimensional image.

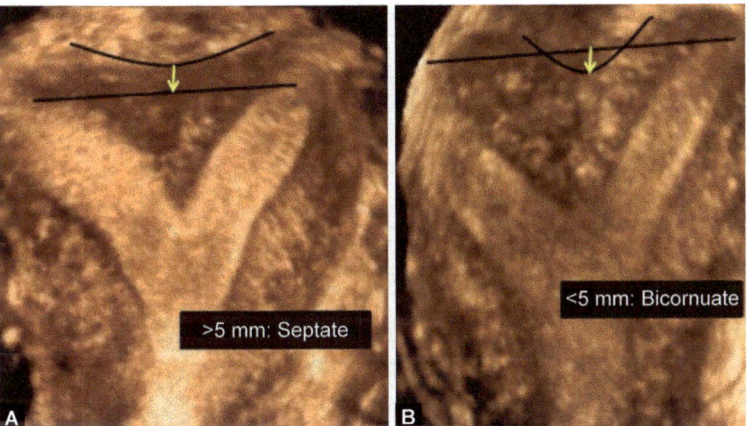

Figs. 7A and B: Septate vs. bicornuate uterus.

(ROI) window is adjusted from fundus to cervix. At this point, the 3D volume is obtained by doing a scan of 90°.

Differentiation between the various subtypes is very important especially between septate and bicornuate as obstetric outcomes are different with each and the treatment approach also varies accordingly. 3D ultrasound is very helpful in differentiating between septate and bicornuate uterus (**Figs. 7 and 8, Table 1**).[20]

Comparative studies with hysteroscopy have shown better results with 3D ultrasound and diagnostic value similar to the MRI with the advantage of lower cost. In 2005, Alcazar et al. compared 3D ultrasound with endoscopy and revealed a sensitivity of 97–100%, positive predictive value of 92%, and negative predictive value of 99% with 96% concordance between US and endoscopy, depending on the type of undiagnosed abnormality.[21] In 2007, Mohamed et al. compared 3D ultrasound with hysteroscopy and laparoscopy, obtaining a sensitivity of 97%, specificity of 96%, positive predictive value of 92%, and negative predictive value of 99%.[22] When specifying the type of malformation, these indices would be up to 92% in the diagnosis of septate uteri and 100% for bicornuate uteri. In a comparative study done with MRI, a Spanish group reports that the images obtained are practically equivalent and in fact, the relationship between the fundus and the uterine cavity can be set perfectly with both ultrasound reconstruction in the coronal plane or coronal sequences obtained with MRI.[23] Many subsequent studies on the classification of uterine morphology also reported high levels of agreement between 3D ultrasound, HSG, and laparoscopy.[24,25]

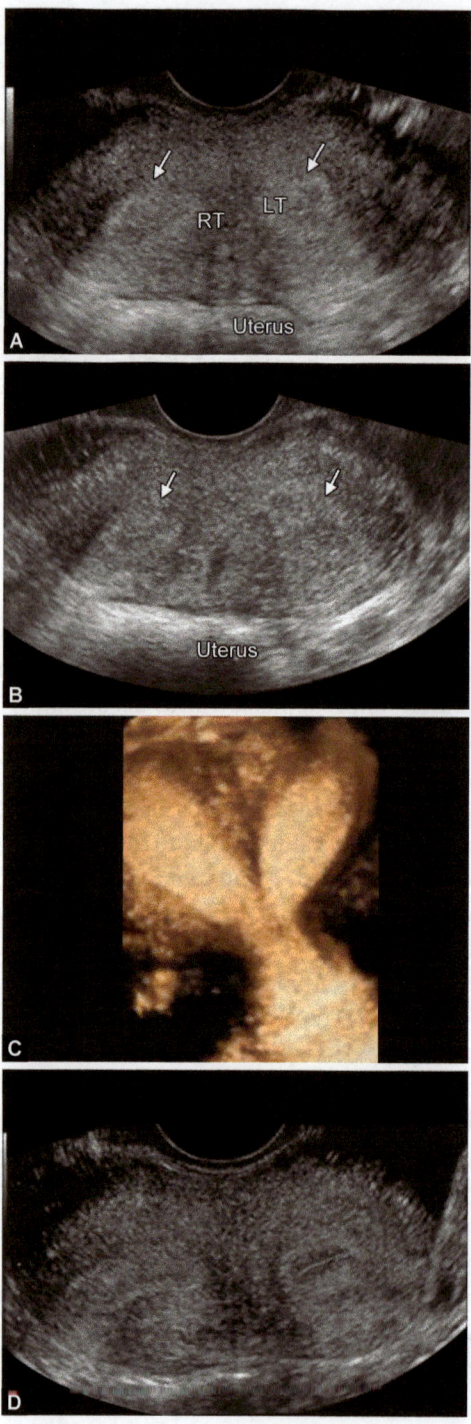

Figs. 8A to D: Two-dimensional and three-dimensional images of a bicornuate uterus.

Table 1: Differences between septate and bicornuate uterus.

Septate	Bicornuate
Angle between two endometrial cavities <75	Angle between two endometrial cavities >75
Linear uterine fundus	Fundus with notch
Distance between horns <4 cm	Distance between horns >4 cm
Distance endometrium-fundus >5 mm	Distance endometrium-fundus <5 mm
Vessels in septum: Yes	Vessels in septum: No

■ CONCLUSION

Ultrasound, especially 3D ultrasound, plays a pivotal role in RPL, both in the evaluation and diagnosis, prognostication and reassuring the woman once she is pregnant about a positive outcome.

■ REFERENCES

1. Reichman DE, Laufer MR. Congenital uterine anomalies affecting reproduction. Best Pract Res Clin Obstet Gyneacol. 2010;24(2):193-208.
2. Pellerito JS, McCarthy SM, Doyle MB, et al. Diagnosis of uterine anomalies: relative accuracy of MR imaging, endovaginal sonography, and hysterosalpingography. Radiology. 1992;183:795-802.
3. Salle B, Sergeant P, Galcherand P, et al. Transvaginal hysterosonographic evaluation of septate uteri: a preliminary report. Hum Reprod. 1996;11:1004-7.
4. The ESHRE Guideline Group on RPL; Atik RB, Christiansen OB, Elson J, et al. ESHRE guideline: recurrent pregnancy loss. Hum Reprod Open. 2018;2018(2).
5. Ayida G, Kennedy S, Barlow D, et al. A comparison of patient tolerance of hysterosalpingo-contrast sonography (HyCoSy) with Echovist-200 and X-ray hysterosalpingography for outpatient investigation of infertile women. Ultrasound Obstet Gynecol. 1996;7:201-4.
6. Jurkovic D, Geipel A, Gruboeck K, et al. Three-dimensional ultrasound for the assessment of uterine anatomy and detection of congenital anomalies: a comparison with hysterosalpingography and two-dimensional sonography. Ultrasound Obstet Gynecol. 1995;5:233-7.
7. Kupesic S, Kurjak A. Septate uterus: detection and prediction of obstetrical complications by different forms of ultrasonography. J Ultrasound Med. 1998;17:631-6.
8. Merz E. Three-dimensional transvaginal ultrasound in gynecological diagnosis. Ultrasound Obstet Gynecol. 1999;14(2):81-6.
9. Abuhamad AZ, Singleton S, Zhao Y, et al. The Z technique: an easy approach to the display of the mid-coronal plane of the uterus in volume sonography. J Ultrasound Med. 2006;25(5):607-12.
10. Saravelos SH, Cocksedge AK, Li TC. Prevalence and diagnosis of congenital uterine anomalies in women with reproductive failure: a critical appraisal. Hum Reprod Update. 2008;14(5):415-29.

11. Ghi T, Casadio P, Kuleva M, et al. Accuracy of three-dimensional ultrasound in diagnosis and classification of congenital uterine anomalies. Fertil Steril. 2009;92(2):808-13.
12. Homer HA, Li TC, Cooke ID. The septate uterus: a review of management and reproductive outcome. Fertil Steril. 2000;73(1):1-14.
13. Salim R, Woelfer B, Backos M, et al. Reproducibility of three-dimensional ultrasound diagnosis of congenital uterine anomalies. Ultrasound Obstet Gynecol. 2003;21(6):578-82.
14. Woelfer B, Salim R, Banerjee S, et al. Reproductive outcomes in women with congenital uterine anomalies detected by three-dimensional ultrasound screening. Obstet Gynecol. 2001;98(6):1099-103.
15. Ford HB, Schust DJ. Recurrent pregnancy loss: etiology, diagnosis, and therapy. Rev Obstet Gynecol. 2009;2(2):76-83.
16. The American Fertility Society classifications of adnexal adhesions, distal tubal occlusion, tubal occlusion secondary to tubal ligation, tubal pregnancies, müllerian anomalies and intrauterine adhesions. Fertil Steril. 1988;49(6):944-55.
17. Troiano RN, McCarthy SM. Mullerian duct anomalies: imaging and clinical issues. Radiology. 2004;233(1):19-34.
18. Grimbizis GF, Gordts S, Di Spiezio Sardo, et al. The ESHRE/ESGE consensus on the classification of female genital tract congenital anomalies. Hum Reprod. 2013;28(8):2032-44.
19. Raga F, Bauset C, Remohi J, et al. Reproductive impact of congenital Müllerian anomalies. Hum Reprod. 1997;12(10):2277-81.
20. Fernando B-M, Noemi M, Mari PE. Uterine malformations: Diagnosis with 3D/4D Ultrasound. Donald School Journal of Ultrasound in Obstetrics and Gynaecology. 2015;3:1-26.
21. Alcázar JL. Three-dimensional ultrasound in Gynaecology: current status and future perspectives. Curr Women's Health Rev. 2005;1:1-14.
22. Mohamed M, Momtaz MD, Alaa N, et al. Three dimensional ultrasonography in the evaluation of uterine cavity. MEFS J. 2007;12:41-6.
23. Bermejo C, Martínez Ten P, Cantarero R, et al. Three-dimensional ultrasound in the diagnosis of Müllerian duct anomalies and concordance with magnetic resonance imaging. Ultrasound in Obstetrics and Gynecology. 2010;35(5):593-601.
24. Chan YY, Jayaprakasan K, Tan A, et al. Reproductive outcomes in women with congenital uterine anomalies: a systematic review. Ultrasound Obstet Gynecol. 2011;38(4):371-82.
25. Practice Committee of the American Society for Reproductive Medicine. Evaluation and treatment of recurrent pregnancy loss: a committee opinion. Fertil Steril. 2012;98(5):1103-11.

Chapter 5
Progesterones in Recurrent Pregnancy Loss

Bharti Dhorepatil, Parzan Mistry

■ INTRODUCTION

Early pregnancy loss or miscarriage is identified in almost 10–15% of all the clinically recognized pregnancies.[1]

The definition of recurrent pregnancy loss (RPL) has long been debated and differs among international societies. For the European Society for Human Reproduction and Embryology (ESHRE)[2] and the Royal College of Obstetricians and Gynaecologists (RCOG),[3] RPL refers to three consecutive pregnancy losses, including nonvisualized ones. However, according to the American Society for Reproductive Medicine (ASRM),[4] it is defined as two or more clinical pregnancy losses (documented by ultrasonography or histopathologic examination) but not necessarily consecutive.

Recurrent spontaneous miscarriage is spontaneous loss of three or more consecutive pregnancies which are less than 20 weeks of gestation. Recurrent miscarriages accounts for 1% of the couples who are attempting to have a child.

It has been seen that increased number of miscarriages increases the chances in the subsequent pregnancies and the percentages vary from 13% to 17% after the first miscarriage to 55% after the third miscarriage.

Unexplained recurrent miscarriage is associated with substantial adverse clinical and psychological consequences for the women and their families.

In many instances, the etiology for recurrent pregnancy losses cannot be pinpointed however it becomes essential for us to find out the cause to help us devise a therapy to reduce miscarriages and have a live healthy baby.

Of the causes of RPL, one of them is inadequate secretion of endogenous progesterone in early pregnancy.

■ PROGESTERONE—THE HORMONE

Progesterone, a female sex hormone, is essential to achieve and maintain a healthy pregnancy. It is secreted naturally by the corpus luteum during the second half of the menstrual cycle and by the corpus luteum and placenta during early pregnancy. It induces secretory changes in the endometrium essential for endometrial maturation, endometrial stabilization, embryo implantation, and proper regulation of inflammatory mediators to create adequate positive immune response in early pregnancy, preventing pregnancy loss.

■ HISTORY OF PROGESTERONE

1933: Allen described the molecular formula of progesterone.

1940: Russel Marker began to synthesize progesterone from diosgenin extracted from Japanese plant *Dioscorea tokoro* and later *Dioscorea mexicana*.

1950: Birch obtained a compound with progestin activity four to eight times higher than progesterone by replacing the methyl group in position 19 with hydrogen atom.

■ PROGESTERONE IN MENSTRUAL CYCLE

Progesterone is essential for the implantation and maintenance of early human pregnancy. The follicular phase of the menstrual cycle is estrogen dominated, while the luteal phase of the menstrual cycle is progesterone dominated.[5]

Secretion of progesterone converts an estrogen-primed proliferative endometrium into a secretory one, which is blastocyst receptive. Before ovulation, granulosa cells in the follicle biosynthesize and secrete estrogen. After follicle rupture and release of the ovum, these granulosa cells mature to form the corpus luteum, which is responsible for secretion of progesterone and estrogen in the latter part of the cycle. If fertilization does not occur within 1 to 2 days, the corpus luteum will continue to enlarge for 10–12 days followed by regression of the gland and concomitant cessation of estrogen and progesterone release. If fertilization occurs, the corpus luteum will continue to grow and function for the first 2 to 3 months of pregnancy. After this time, it will slowly regress as the placenta assumes the role of hormonal biosynthesis for the maintenance of pregnancy.[6]

■ PROGESTERONE IN OVARIAN CYCLE BASED ON "TWO-CELL TWO-GONADOTROPIN THEORY"

This theory establishes that ovarian steroids are synthesized from cholesterol through the interactions of theca and granulosa cells **(Fig. 1)**.

Theca cells: Luteinizing hormone (LH) binds to luteinizing/chorionic gonadotropin receptor (LH/CGR) on the cell surface and stimulates the expression of the steroidogenic enzymes necessary for androgen production. Cholesterol is mobilized into mitochondria by steroidogenic acute regulatory protein (STAR) where it is converted to pregnenolone by cholesterol side chain cleavage enzyme (CYP11A1). Pregnenolone diffuses into the smooth

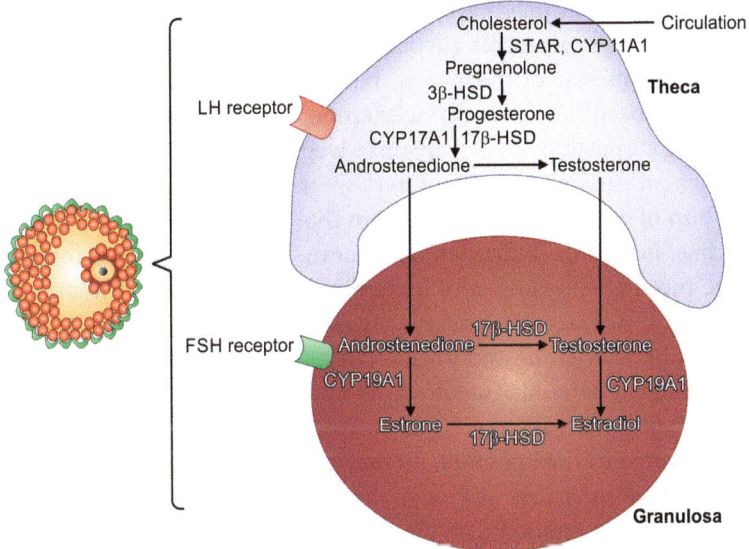

Fig. 1: Progesterone in ovarian cycle.
Source: Häggström M, Richfield D. Diagram of the pathways of human steroidogenesis. Wiki J Med. 2014;1(1).

endoplasmic reticulum and is converted to progesterone by 3β-hydroxysteroid dehydrogenase (3βHSD). Progesterone is then converted to androstenedione by 17α-hydroxylase/17,20 desmolase (CYP17A1).

Granulosa cells: Follicle-stimulating hormone (FSH) via signaling through follicle-stimulating hormone receptor (FSHR) stimulates the expression of enzymes necessary for estrogen synthesis. Androstenedione produced by theca cells diffuses into granulosa cells and is converted to testosterone by the enzyme 17β-hydroxysteroid dehydrogenase (HSD17B) or to estrone by aromatase (CYP19A1). CYP19A1 utilizes testosterone to produce 17β-estradiol. However, HSD17B can also produce 17β-estradiol using estrone as a substrate.

ROLE OF PROGESTERONE IN LUTEAL PHASE AND RATIONALE BEHIND USING IT FOR THE LUTEAL PHASE SUPPORT

- The use of gonadotropin-releasing hormone (GnRH) agonists into ovarian stimulation protocols in in-vitro fertilization (IVF) became associated with improved outcomes. Pituitary function does not resume completely until 2–3 weeks after the end of GnRH-agonist therapy; however, luteal phase support was considered essential to counter any luteal insufficiency that may have a negative impact on an early pregnancy. Most treatment protocols advocate the use of progesterone throughout the first trimester of pregnancy, based on the findings of Shamma et al., who used 17-hydroxyprogesterone as a marker to demonstrate ongoing corpus luteum activity up to week 10 of pregnancy.[7] This finding confirmed earlier estimates of 8-10 weeks.[8,9] Progesterone is given with the aim of assisting a corpus luteum that may have been compromised during ovulation induction or oocyte retrieval. GnRH-antagonists have recently appeared with increasing frequency in ART treatment. In contrast to the agonist, antagonists are administered for a significantly shorter period of time and have a shorter duration of effect. Their impact on the corpus luteum is unknown and merits further study. Progesterone support of the luteal phase (up to the serum pregnancy test) in IVF cycles is supported by the literature, though support beyond the pregnancy test may not be indicated. Although serum progesterone levels are higher after IM administration than after vaginal administration, the pregnancy rates after these two types of support are comparable. The world's largest phase III study called Lotus I and Lotus II is ongoing in several European, Middle East, and Asian countries to assess the role of dydrogesterone, micronized progesterone vaginal tablets, and micronized progesterone gel as progesterone support in artificial reproductive techniques, including IVF. Based on the available clinical data, progesterone support (vaginal micronized progesterone and dydrogesterone) is beneficial in women presenting with a clinical diagnosis of threatened miscarriage with relative risk reduction in the miscarriage rate of 47% with the use of progesterone.

■ ROLE OF PROGESTERONE IN RPL: WHAT DOES COCHRANE HAVE TO SAY?

Cochrane in 2017 searched for evidences and identified a total of 13 trials that enrolled a total of 2,556 women with history of recurrent miscarriages. These trials found that giving progestogen medication to women with recurrent miscarriages early in their pregnancy may help lower the rates of miscarriage in that pregnancy from 26.3% to 19.4%.

Studies taken into consideration:
- The miscarriage rate was lower in women with RPL receiving progesterone treatment, compared to placebo (OR 0.39; 95% CI 021-0.72) (Haas and Ramsey 2013).
- A more recent double blind, placebo-controlled, randomized trial of oral dydrogesterone (given from the time that a live fetus was confirmed by ultrasound until 20 weeks of gestation) among 360 women with a RPL also showed a benefit of progesterone in reducing a subsequent risk of

miscarriage compared with placebo (RR 2.4; 95% CI 1.3-5.9) (Kumar et al. 2014).

- In a study conducted by Coomarasamy et al. in 2015, a total of 802 women receiving progesterone and 784 receiving placebo, women with RPL who were randomized to the intervention group had a lower risk of subsequent pregnancy loss (RR 0.72; 95% CI 0.53-0.97) and higher live birth rate (RR 1.07; 95% CI 1.02-1.15) compared with those who did not. Most of these trials had evidence of moderate quality. It was found out that progestogen treatment may be most helpful for women who had had at least three miscarriages before they started the study. It was also found out that the route of progesterone administration (oral, vaginal, sublingual or injectable) did not affect the outcome.

■ THE PROMISE STUDY

The PROMISE study was designed to test the hypothesis that in women with unexplained recurrent miscarriage, progesterone (400 mg vaginal capsules, twice daily), started as soon as practicable after a positive urinary pregnancy test (and no later than 6 weeks of gestation) and continued to 12 weeks of gestation, compared with placebo, would increase live births beyond 24 completed weeks of pregnancy by at least 10% **(Fig. 2)**. A total of 1,568

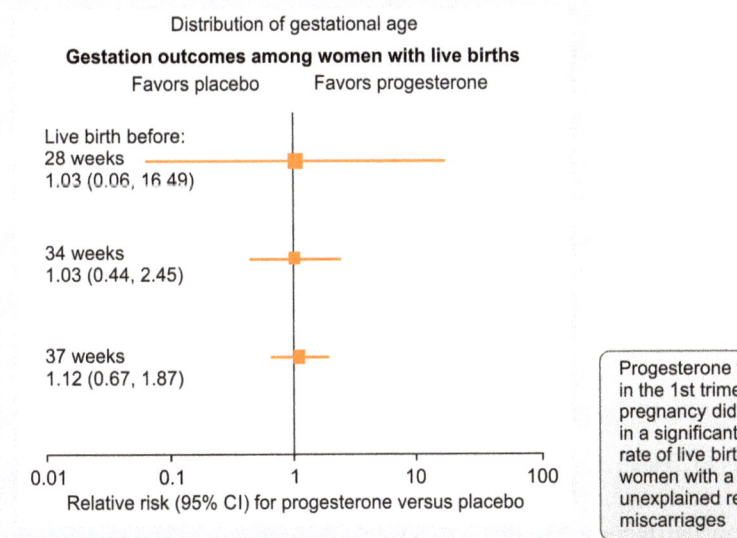

Fig. 2: PROMISE trial—conclusion.
Source: Coomarasamy A, Williams H, Truchanowicz E, et al. A randomized trial of progesterone in women with recurrent miscarriages. New Eng J Med. 2015;373(22):2141-8.

participants were screened for eligibility. Of the 836 women randomized, 404 participants received progesterone therapy and 432 received placebo. The follow-up rate for the primary outcome was 826 out of 836 (98.8%). The live birth rate in the progesterone group was 65.8% (262/398), and in the placebo group it was 63.3% (271/428), giving a relative risk (RR) of 1.04 [95% confidence interval (CI) 0.94 to 1.15; p = 0.45]. The PROMISE trial is the largest clinical trial ever conducted on the subject of RPL. The trial was adequately sized and methodologically robust to conclude that vaginal progesterone therapy in the first trimester of pregnancy in women with RM is of no benefit and, therefore, should not be used in clinical settings. Future work could investigate the effectiveness of progesterone therapy during the luteal phase of the menstrual cycle, or for patients who have threatened miscarriage.

The argument for use of progesterone (vaginal micronized progesterone and dydrogesterone) is that there is no evidence of harm and some evidence of benefit, although not coming from huge multicentric trials. The decision should be based on clinician's discretion until strong evidence is available to recommend routine use. The doses of progesterone that are generally used in clinical practice for recurrent miscarriage as per current evidence are as follows:

- Oral dydrogesterone 10 mg BD till 20 weeks of pregnancy.
- *Micronized progesterone*: 400 mg/day vaginally till 20 weeks of pregnancy.

■ INTERNATIONAL GUIDELINES

RCOG (2011) and ESHRE (2017) guidelines for recurrent miscarriages also state that the use of vaginal progesterone does not improve the live birth rates in women with unexplained RPL.

Royal Australian and New Zealand College of Obstetrics and Gynaecologists (2013) state that progesterone may reduce the risk but cannot be recommended based on current evidence.

FOGSI position statement (2015): No evidence of harm and some evidence of benefit, although not coming from huge multicentric trials. Decision of starting progesterone should be based on clinician's discretion, until that time strong evidence is available to recommend routine use.

Yale University Study

According to researchers at the Yale School of Medicine and University of Illinois at Chicago, progesterone could give hope to women who suffer multiple miscarriages in the first 4 to 5 weeks of pregnancy. The researchers revealed that intrauterine fetal demise (IUFD) currently affects approximately 30,000 women each year in the US, while 25% of all women who become pregnant suffer a loss in the first trimester.

However, some women suffer a loss every time they are pregnant. The researchers went about studying the effects of micronized plant-derived progesterone in 116 women who had experienced two or more pregnancy losses up to that point.

The researchers used the endometrial function test (EFT), which was created by study coauthor Dr Harvey Kliman, Director of the Reproductive and Placental Research Unit in the Yale Department of Obstetrics, Gynecology, and Reproductive Sciences, in order to determine whether a woman's endometrium is healthy and can sustain the embryo.

According to the researchers, an abnormal EFT is associated with pregnancy failure, while a normal EFT is associated with a successful pregnancy. They prescribed progesterone 2 days after ovulation to women in the study with an abnormal nCyclinE molecular marker level. It is at this time when the uterine lining matures in preparation for a potential pregnancy. The researchers said they believe that the progesterone caused the patients' endometrium to produce more endometrial secretions which furthermore suggest that progesterone helps increase implantation rates in people with recurrent miscarriages.

■ A RANDOMIZED TRIAL OF PROGESTERONE IN EARLY PREGNANCY: A ONE OF ITS TRIAL BY ARRI COOMARASAMY ET AL

In women who had one or two miscarriages, 76% of those given progesterone went on to have a live birth, compared with 72% of the placebo group. Among women who had three or more miscarriages, 72% of those given progesterone went on to have a live birth, compared with 52% of the placebo group. Women were randomly assigned to receive vaginal suppositories containing either 400 mg of progesterone or matching placebo twice daily, from the time at which they presented with bleeding through 16 weeks of gestation. The primary outcome was the birth of a live born baby after at least 34 weeks of gestation.

A total of 4,153 women, recruited at 48 hospitals in the United Kingdom, were randomly assigned to receive progesterone (2,079 women) or placebo (2,074 women). The percentage of women with available data for the primary outcome was 97% (4,038 of 4,153 women). The incidence of live births after at least 34 weeks of gestation was 75% (1,513 of 2,025 women) in the progesterone group and 72% (1,459 of 2,013 women) in the placebo group (relative rate: 1.03; 95% confidence interval [CI], 1.00–1.07; $P = 0.08$). The sensitivity analysis, in which missing primary outcome data were imputed, resulted in a similar finding (relative rate: 1.03; 95% CI, 1.00–1.07; $P = 0.08$). The incidence of adverse events did not differ significantly between the groups.

Among women with bleeding in early pregnancy, progesterone therapy administered during the first trimester did not result in a significantly higher incidence of live births than placebo.

■ CONCLUSION

Though most of the national guidelines and Cochrane analysis suggest that there is no proven role of routine use of progesterone in patients with recurrent miscarriages, the recent paper of Arri Coomarasamy et al. has changed the perspectives of the clinicians when they concluded in one of the largest trials of its kind that progesterone when administered in patients with recurrent miscarriages increased the chances of live birth rates in these patients. Since the use of progesterone has not known any adverse effects in the patients, considering the recent studies it may be worth trying out in patients with recurrent pregnancy losses.[10]

■ REFERENCES

1. Practice Committee of the American Society for Reproductive Medicine. Evaluation and treatment of recurrent pregnancy loss: a committee opinion. Fertil Steril. 2012;98(5):1103-11.
2. Kolte AM, Bernardi LA, Christiansen OB, et al. Early pregnancy. Hum Reprod. 2015;30(3):495-8.
3. Royal College of Obstetricians and Gynaecologists. Scientific Advisory Committee, Guideline No. 17. (2011). The Investigation and treatment of couples with recurrent t First trimester and Second-trimester miscarriage. [online] Available from https://www.rcog.org.uk/globalassets/documents/guidelines/gtg_17.pdf [Last accessed November, 2019].
4. Evaluation and treatment of recurrent pregnancy loss: a committee opinion. Practice Committee of the American Society for Reproductive Medicine. Fertil Steril. 2012;98(5):1103-11.
5. Cameron IT, Irvine G, Norman JE. Menstruation. In: Hiller SJ, Kitchener HC, Neilson JP (Eds). Scientific Essentials of Reproductive Medicine. London: WB Saunders, 1996.
6. Graham JD, Clarke CL. Physiological action of progesterone in target tissues. Endocrine Reviews. 1997;18(4):502-19.
7. Shamma FN, Penzias AS, Thatcher S, et al. Corpus luteum function in successful in vitro fertilization cycles. Fertil Steril. 1992;57(5):1107-9.
8. Yoshimi T, Strott CA, Marshall JR, et al. Corpus luteum function in early pregnancy. J Clin Endocrinol Metab.1969;29(2):225-30.
9. Tulchinsky D, Hobel CJ. Plasma human chorionic gonadotropin, estrone, estradiol, estriol, progesterone, and 17 alpha-hydroxyprogesterone in human pregnancy. 3. Early normal pregnancy. Am J Obstet Gynecol. 1973;117(7): 884-93.
10. Coomarasamy A, Dewall AJ, Cheed V, et al. A randomized trial of progesterone with women with bleeding in early pregnancy. New Eng J Med. 2019;380: 1815-24.

Chapter 6: Antiphospholipids in Recurrent Pregnancy Loss

Bhaskar Pal, Tulika Jha

■ INTRODUCTION

Antiphospholipid syndrome (APS or APLS) is an autoimmune, hypercoagulable disorder caused by antiphospholipid (aPL) antibodies. It provokes arterial and venous thrombosis and is associated with pregnancy complications, including recurrent pregnancy loss (RPL), preeclampsia, thrombosis, autoimmune thrombocytopenia, fetal growth restriction, and fetal loss. It is the most important treatable cause of RPL.

Women with the clinical features of APS should be tested for *three antiphospholipid antibodies* that have proven association with the diagnosis of APS: *lupus anticoagulant (LAC), anticardiolipin (aCL) antibody, and anti-beta-2 glycoprotein I antibody*.

Antiphospholipid syndrome is classified as primary or secondary, depending on its association with other autoimmune disorders.

- *Primary APS*: It is diagnosed in patients demonstrating the clinical and laboratory criteria for the disease without other recognized autoimmune disease.
- *Secondary APS*: It is diagnosed in patients with other autoimmune disorders, such as systemic lupus erythematosus (SLE).

Catastrophic APS: APS may rarely lead to generalized thrombosis which may cause multiorgan failure and death. This clinical condition is known as "catastrophic antiphospholipid syndrome" (CAPS).

■ EPIDEMIOLOGY

Antiphospholipid antibodies are present in about 15% of the women with RPL and in only 2% of the women with a low risk obstetric history.

In the United States, women have been reported to account for approximately 80% of patients with APS and they predominantly belong to the reproductive age group (15-50 years). This is similar to other autoimmune states.

The aPL antibodies account for 65-70% of cases of venous thrombosis in women with venous thrombosis in unusual sites (e.g. cerebral, portal, splenic, subclavian, and mesenteric veins). The aPL antibodies are detected in approximately 2% of all patients with nontraumatic venous thrombosis.

Approximately 24% of thrombotic events have been found to occur during pregnancy or the postpartum period. The rate for thrombosis or stroke is 5–12%. These observations suggest that women with documented APS should not take estrogen–progestin combination oral contraceptives.

■ HISTORY

The "International Consensus Statement for the Diagnosis of Antiphospholipid Syndrome," published in 1999 by Wilson et al., serves as a set of criteria similar to that for the diagnosis of other autoimmune disorders. It is known as the *Sapporo criteria*.[1] The criteria were updated in 2006 by Miyakis et al. to reflect new insights into APS and are known as the *Sydney criteria*.[2]

According to these criteria, the diagnosis requires that the patient have *at least one clinical and one laboratory criterion.*

Clinical Criteria

The clinical criteria for APS include the following:
- One or more clinical episodes of arterial, venous, or small-vessel thrombosis, occurring within any tissue or organ.
- One or more unexplained deaths of morphologically normal fetuses at or after 10 weeks' gestation.
- One or more premature births of morphologically normal fetuses at or before 34 weeks' gestation because of eclampsia or severe preeclampsia or features consistent with placental insufficiency.
- Three or more consecutive, unexplained spontaneous abortions before 10 weeks' gestation, with maternal anatomic or hormonal abnormalities and paternal and maternal chromosomal causes excluded.

According to the Royal College of Obstetricians and Gynaecologists (RCOG) guidelines on recurrent miscarriage (GTG 17), the adverse pregnancy outcomes which should be present to fulfill the clinical criteria are similar:[3]
- Three or more consecutive miscarriages before 10 weeks of gestation.
- One or more morphologically normal fetal losses after the 10th week of gestation.
- One or more preterm births before the 34th week of gestation owing to placental disease.

Laboratory Criteria

Criteria for laboratory testing, which are consistent with current clinical management guidelines from the American Congress of Obstetricians and Gynecologists (ACOG), include the following:
- *Anticardiolipin antibodies*: Anticardiolipin IgG or IgM antibodies present at moderate or high levels (i.e. >40 GPL or MPL or >99th percentile) in the blood on two or more occasions at least 12 weeks' apart.

- *Anti-beta 2-glycoprotein I antibodies IgG or IgM*: In titers above the 99th percentile for normal as defined by the laboratory performing the test, on two or more occasions at least 12 weeks' apart.
- *Lupus anticoagulant*: LAC detected in the blood on two or more occasions at least 12 weeks' apart, according to the guidelines of the International Society on Thrombosis and Hemostasis.

Lupus anticoagulant is tested by indirect methods, i.e. by activated partial thromboplastin time (APTT), Kaolin clotting time (KCT) or dilute Russell Viper Venom test (DRVVT), the latter being the most reliable.

■ RISK FACTORS

The risk factors for developing APS include:
- *Primary APS:* Genetic marker HLA-DR7
- *Secondary APS:*
  - SLE or other autoimmune disorders
  - *Genetic markers:* HLA-B8, HLA-DR2, HLA-DR3
  - *Race:* Blacks, Hispanics, Asians, Native Americans.

A "two-hit" theory has been proposed according to which a second risk factor (age, hypertension, diabetes, obesity, smoking, pregnancy, surgery, and other genetic hypercoagulable state) incites the thrombotic effects of aPL.

■ ETIOLOGY

Like other autoimmune disorders, APS does not have a known etiology. It is known, though, that the passive transfer of maternal antibodies mediates autoimmune disorders in the fetus and newborn. The mechanism of excess autoantibody production and immune complex formation is not well understood.

- *Genetic*: Certain genetic factors may be important, as indicated by a number of family and twin studies for SLE and the demonstration of an increased frequency of HLA-DR2, HLA-DR3, and HLA-DR4 null alleles in patients with SLE.
- *Infection*: During infectious disease processes, including viral [e.g. HIV, Epstein-Barr virus (EBV), cytomegalovirus (CMV), adenoviruses], bacterial (e.g. bacterial endocarditis, tuberculosis, *Mycoplasma pneumonia*), spirochetal (e.g. syphilis, leptospirosis, Lyme disease), and parasitic (e.g. malaria infection) infections, cell damage occurs and there is disruption of cellular membranes. The phospholipids (PL), which are ubiquitous in nature and are present on the inner surface of the cell membrane and intracellular organelles, are consequently released. These disruptive processes release aPL antibodies.

- *Epitope mimicry in autoimmune disease*: Some protein databases and sequences show high homology between the hexapeptides that bind to ILA-1, ILA-3, and H-3 mAbs and the membrane particles of different bacteria and viruses, e.g. *Haemophilus influenzae, Neisseria gonorrhoeae,* and *Shigella dysenteriae,* EBV, HIV, etc. This epitope mimicry may propagate the autoimmune status.
- Drugs and vaccines associated with APS include the following: procainamide, quinidine, propranolol, hydralazine, phenytoin, chlorpromazine, interferon alfa, quinine, amoxicillin, and tetanus toxoid.

■ PATHOPHYSIOLOGY

Studies on patients with lupus erythematous have shown association between aPL antibodies and particular human leukocyte antigen (HLA) alleles and HLA-linked epitopes (e.g. HLA-DR7, HLA-DR4). The HLA-DR3 phenotypes seem to predispose to the formation of aCL antibodies and antinuclear antibodies (ANAs), but this has not been confirmed in patients.

The aPL antibodies namely aCL, LAC, anti-b2GP1, bind to anionic proteins of the plasma membranes, thereby causing an autoimmune reaction and complement activation. The antibodies also interact with different factors of the coagulation cascade thereby activating it. LAC antibodies bind to prothrombin, thus increasing its cleavage to thrombin, its active form.

The biologic effects mediated by the human aPL antibodies include the following:
- Reactivity with endothelial structures that disturbs the balance of prostaglandin E2/thromboxane production.
- Interaction with platelet PLs, with consequent upregulation of platelet aggregation.
- Dysregulation of complement activation.
- Interaction of aPLs with phosphatidyl serine exposed during trophoblast syncytium formation, which raises the possibility of a more direct effect of these autoantibodies on placental structures.

In patients with primary APS, the presence of the 3 aCL isotypes plus LAC has been associated with a higher number of recurrent spontaneous abortions, compared with other possible combinations of aCL isotypes.

■ CLINICAL FEATURES

The clinical features associated with APS can be categorized as—(1) obstetric and (2) nonobstetric features.
The obstetric features are as follows:
- Unexplained fetal death or stillbirth
- Recurrent pregnancy loss—three or more spontaneous abortions with no more than one live birth

- Unexplained second or third trimester fetal death
- Severe preeclampsia at less than 34 weeks' gestation
- Unexplained severe fetal growth restriction
- Chorea gravidarum.

The nonobstetric features of APS are as follows:
- Nontraumatic thrombosis or thromboembolism (venous or arterial)
- Stroke, especially in individuals aged 24–50 years
- Unexplained transient ischemic attack
- Unexplained amaurosis fugax
- Autoimmune thrombocytopenia
- Autoimmune hemolytic anemia
- Unexplained prolongation of a clotting assay
- Livedo reticularis
- SLE or other connective tissue disorder
- False-positive serologic test result for syphilis.

COMPLICATIONS

Maternal

- Fetal loss which is often due to placenta-mediated complications in women with pure obstetric APS (OAPS).
- Women with APS have an increased incidence of preeclampsia, which frequently develops prior to 34 weeks' gestation and is of a severe degree. The incidence of severe preeclampsia requiring premature delivery is also increased.
- Preterm delivery, either spontaneous or induced due to severe preeclampsia.
- Antiphospholipid syndrome is one of the major causes of thrombosis and its complications in women, with arterial thrombosis, coronary artery occlusions, and venous thrombosis being reported in patients with this syndrome. Previous thrombosis in the face of a diagnosis of APS has been documented to have a recurrence rate of 25% per year in untreated patients.
- Morbidity may also be associated with anticoagulation in patients treated with heparin or low-molecular-weight heparins in pregnancy.
- Antiphospholipid syndrome is also associated with infertility and pregnancy complications, such as spontaneous abortions, prematurity, and stillbirths.
- Landry-Guillain-Barré-Strohl syndrome (LGBSS) is an acute inflammatory demyelinating polyradiculoneuropathy, although exceedingly rare in pregnancy, can occur in patients with APS and lupus. Patients usually present with progressive bilateral and symmetrical muscle weakness accompanied by mild sensory symptoms, including paresthesia, numbness, and tingling. The disease can progress to involve

the respiratory muscles, resulting in respiratory failure. Two-thirds of the patients have a history of viral-like infections, especially CMV, 1–3 weeks' prior to the onset of symptoms.
- There is an additional elevated risk of adrenal gland bleeds leading to Waterhouse-Friderichsen syndrome (*Neisseria meningitidis* caused primary adrenal insufficiency). This will require adrenal steroid replacement treatment for life.
- Mortality rates during pregnancy are not well characterized. Multiorgan failure has been described during pregnancy by Asherson and during postpartum by Kochenour.

Perinatal

- *Perinatal morbidity*: The morbidity and mortality may be influenced by indicated preterm delivery for maternal severe preeclampsia or fetal growth restriction.
- Neonatal lupus dermatitis, a variety of systemic and hematologic abnormalities, and isolated congenital heart block have been associated with APS and SLE.
- *Perinatal mortality*: Fetal deaths at or beyond 20 weeks' gestation may be attributable to APS involvement. The rate of fetal loss may exceed 90% in untreated patients with APS.

■ DIFFERENTIAL DIAGNOSES

Antiphospholipid syndrome needs to be differentiated from the following clinical conditions:
- Disseminated intravascular coagulation
- Infective endocarditis
- Thrombotic thrombocytopenic purpura (TTP).

■ INVESTIGATIONS

The following laboratory tests should be considered in a patient suspected of having APS:
- aCL antibodies (IgG, IgM)
- Anti-beta-2 glycoprotein I antibodies (IgG, IgM)
- LA tests such as DRVVT
- Activated partial thromboplastin time (aPTT)
- Serologic test for syphilis (false-positive result)
- CBC count (thrombocytopenia, hemolytic anemia).

Lupus Anticoagulant

An abnormal LA finding is the laboratory test result that confers the strongest risk for thrombosis. LA is directed against plasma coagulation molecules. In vitro, this interaction results in the paradoxical prolongation of clotting assays, such as clotting time, aPTT, KCT, and DRVVT. A threshold of approximately 1.6 for the DRVVT ratio has been recommended for helping discriminate APS from non-APS.

Anticardiolipin Antibodies

Enzyme-linked immunosorbent assay (ELISA) is currently the test of choice. Of the three known isotypes of aCL (i.e., IgG, IgM, IgA), IgG correlates most strongly with thrombotic events. The reference range findings are as follows:
- Less than 15 immunoglobulin G (IgG) phospholipids units (GPL): Absent or none detected
- Less than 12 immunoglobulin M (IgM) phospholipids units (MPL): Absent or none detected
- Less than 12 immunoglobulin A (IgA) phospholipids units (APL): Absent or none detected.

Anti-β_2 Glycoprotein-1 Antibodies

ELISA is the test used to detect these antibodies, IgM and IgG isotypes. As per the APS diagnostic criteria, these anti-β_2 glycoprotein-1 antibodies of IgG and/or IgM isotype should be present in the plasma, in a titer greater than the 99th percentile to be considered a positive test result.

Cardiolipin is the dominant antigen used in most serologic tests for syphilis; consequently, these patients may have a false-positive test result for syphilis.

There is considerable interlaboratory variation in the aPL estimation. The results may also vary in the same woman over time, due to presence of infections, suboptimal sample collection, and lack of standard results in many laboratories (RCOG GTG).

Currently, there is much investigation into risk-stratifying patients based on aPL profile, aPL titers, associated autoimmune disease, and other cardiovascular risk factors. "Triple-positive" patients (LA, anti-beta-2 glycoprotein antibodies, AC antibodies) are at highest risk for thrombosis or abnormal pregnancy, and possibly for recurrence. Standardized scoring systems such as the Global Antiphospholipid Syndrome Score (GAPSS) are being developed.

■ IMAGING

Imaging studies are helpful for confirming a thrombotic event. Examples are the use of computed tomography (CT) or magnetic resonance imaging (MRI) scans of the following: brain (for stroke), chest (for pulmonary embolism), and abdomen (for Budd-Chiari syndrome).

Doppler ultrasound studies are recommended for possible detection of deep vein thrombosis.

Two-dimensional echocardiography findings may demonstrate asymptomatic valve thickening, vegetations, or valvular insufficiency.

■ HISTOLOGY

Unlike inflammatory autoimmune diseases, histologic studies of skin or other involved tissue reveal a noninflammatory bland thrombosis with no signs of perivascular inflammation or leukocytoclastic vasculitis. Similarly, biopsy samples from affected kidneys demonstrate glomerular and small arterial microthrombi.

■ TREATMENT

Pregnant women with APS are considered high-risk obstetric patients, and medical care is instituted with this in mind.

In patients receiving or recently treated with corticosteroid therapy, administer supplementation to cover the labor or cesarean delivery.

Pregnancy in itself is not harmful to the mother or the baby unless added work related to the newborn, as well as emotional stress in the family, proves to be too much for a particular patient. Therapeutic abortions are generally not indicated in pregnant women with autoimmune disease.

Obstetric Care

Patients should be counseled in all cases regarding symptoms of thrombosis and thromboembolism and should be educated regarding, and examined frequently for, the signs or symptoms of thrombosis or thromboembolism, severe preeclampsia, or decreased fetal movement.

Ultrasonography is recommended every 3-4 weeks starting at 18-20 weeks' gestation, in patients with a poor obstetric history, evidence of preeclampsia, or evidence of fetal growth restriction.

Human chorionic gonadotropin (hCG) values in the first trimester can be followed to evaluate the viability of the pregnancy. If hCG levels are increasing normally (i.e., doubling every 2 days) in the first month of pregnancy, a successful outcome is predicted in 80-90% of cases. However, when the increases are abnormal (i.e., slower), a poor outcome is predicted in 70-80% of cases.

In patients with uncomplicated APS, ultrasonography is recommended at 30-32 weeks' gestation to assess fetal growth. Lagging fetal growth may reflect uteroplacental insufficiency in patients with APS.

Drugs such as chloroquine and cytotoxic agents are not recommended during pregnancy; patients should stop taking these drugs several months prior to becoming pregnant.

Splenectomy during the early second trimester or at the time of cesarean delivery may be considered in patients with thrombocytopenia refractory to glucocorticoid therapy.

Anticoagulation Therapy

Anticoagulation is the main stay of management in women with RPL and APS.[4] The drugs used are:
- *Low dose aspirin (LDA)*: Heparin.
- *Unfractionated heparin (UFH) or low molecular weight heparin (LMWH)*: Intravenous immunoglobulin (IVIG) or corticosteroids have also been tried, but there is a lack of evidence regarding their benefit in pregnancy outcome.

History of Previous Thrombotic Event

- Full anticoagulation is advised in such women. UFH is recommended in APS and pregnancy with a history of a thromboembolic event. The usual dose is 15,000–20,000 units daily in 2–3 divided doses. The target aPTT is 1.5 times the normal value.
- Low-molecular-weight heparin may also be used in these patients.
- *Dose*: 1 mg/kg 12 hourly or 1.5 mg/kg daily.
- This should be continued till 6 weeks postpartum.

History of Previous Fetal Loss or Premature Delivery (No Previous Thrombotic Event)

Pregnant women with APS should be considered for anticoagulation with LDA and heparin to prevent further miscarriage. A meta-analysis of RCTs reported that the only treatment or treatment combination that leads to a significant increase in the live birth rate among women with APS is LDA plus UFH. This treatment combination significantly reduces the miscarriage rate by 54% (aspirin plus unfractionated heparin compared with aspirin alone: RR 0.46, 95% CI 0.29–0.71). Studies have shown no differences in the efficacy and safety profile of LMWH and UFH.

It is important, though, to counsel the patient regarding potential adverse effects of heparin namely bleeding episodes, hypersensitivity reactions, thrombocytopenia, and osteoporosis. Heparin-induced osteoporosis occurs in 1–2% of cases. Initiation of heparin in the face of a failing pregnancy should be undertaken with caution due to bleeding risks. Heparin does not cross the placenta and, therefore, does not cause any teratogenicity or bleeding manifestations in the fetus. Low molecular weight heparin is as safe as UFH and causes less thrombocytopenia and osteoporosis.

Bone density studies should be considered in patients receiving anticoagulation therapy with heparin or LMWH due to the risks of osteopenia. This may be most important in women who have been treated in a previous pregnancy or are planning pregnancy.

Pregnancies associated with antiphospholipid antibodies and treated with aspirin and heparin benefit substantially in terms of live birth rate of women with recurrent miscarriage, but these pregnancies remain at high risk of complications during all three trimesters, including repeated miscarriage, preeclampsia, fetal growth restriction, and preterm birth: this necessitates careful antenatal surveillance.[5]

- Neither corticosteroids nor IVIG therapy improve the live birth rate of women with recurrent miscarriage associated with antiphospholipid antibodies compared with other treatment modalities; their use may provoke significant maternal and fetal morbidity namely premature delivery, increased rates of neonatal intensive care unit admission, preeclampsia, gestational diabetes, and lower birth weights.
- In APS and RPL, aspirin and heparin are still recommended and aspirin should be started as soon as pregnancy test is positive.
- ACOG and ESHRE guidelines[6] suggest that heparin or LMWH (Enoxaparin 40 mg/day) can be started when UPT is positive while RCOG guidelines suggest same but only when FH is seen on TVS.

■ MANAGEMENT DURING LABOR AND DELIVERY

- Deliver at term
- *Adjust prophylactic anticoagulant dose*: Antithrombotics should be stopped if bleeding starts or patient goes into spontaneous labor. Last injection should be given 12 hours prior to elective CS or induction of labor (IOL).
- *Adjust therapeutic anticoagulant dose*: Stop LMWH 24 hours prior to elective CS or IOL and IV UFH 2-4 hours prior to anticipated delivery in women at high risk of thrombosis.
- Continuous electronic fetal monitoring (EFM) should be done in labor.
- Epidural anesthetic is not recommended if the mother has a marked drop in the maternal platelet count. The use of forceps or the vacuum extractor should be individualized.

Postnatal Management

- Resume anticoagulation 4-6 hours after vaginal delivery and 8-12 hours after CS.
- Women with prior thrombosis should receive prophylaxis for 6 weeks.
- Women without prior thrombosis prophylaxis for 10 days (RCOG) or 6 weeks (ACOG).

- Warfarin is safe during lactation and may be substituted for heparin during the postpartum period to limit further risk of heparin-induced osteoporosis and bone fracture.
- No evidence indicates adverse effects related to breastfeeding, although breastfeeding is not recommended if high doses of cytotoxic or immunosuppressive agents are required.
- Estrogen containing OC should be avoided.

CONCLUSION

Antiphospholipid antibody syndrome is a proved cause for RPL in a selected group of patients. Evaluation for the condition and appropriate treatment will definitely be of benefit.

REFERENCES

1. Wilson WA, Gharavi AE, Koike T, et al. International consensus statement on preliminary classification criteria for definite antiphospholipid syndrome: report of an international workshop. Arthritis & Rheumatism: Official Journal of the American College of Rheumatology. 1999;42(7):1309-11.
2. Miyakis S, Lockshin MD, Atsumi T, et al. International Consensus Statement on an Update of the Classification Criteria for definite antiphospholipid syndrome (APS). J Thromb Haemost. 2006;4(2):295-306.
3. Royal College of Obstetricians and Gynaecologists. Scientific Advisory Committee, Guideline No. 17. (2011). The Investigation and treatment of couples with recurrent First-trimester and Second-trimester miscarriage. [online] Available from https://www.rcog.org.uk/globalassets/documents/guidelines/gtg_17.pdf [Last accessed November, 2019].
4. de Jong PG, Goddijn M, Middeldorp S. Antithrombotic therapy for pregnancy loss. Hum Reprod Update. 2013;19(6):656-73.
5. Tong M, Viall CA, Chamley LW. Antiphospholipid antibodies and the placenta: a systematic review of their in vitro effects and modulation by treatment. Hum Reprod Update. 2014;21(1):97-118.
6. Loss RP. Guideline of the European Society of Human Reproduction and Embryology. ESHRE Early Pregnancy Guidline Development Group. 2017.

Chapter 7: Heparin in Recurrent Pregnancy Loss

Sujata Misra, Charmila Ayyavoo

■ INTRODUCTION

Recurrent pregnancy loss (RPL) is the loss of three or more pregnancies at ≤20 weeks or have a fetal weight <500 g. The incidence is around 1% in fertile families. Many of them are embryonic losses which occur early and the rest are anembryonic which can occur after 14 weeks of pregnancy.[1] A couple suffering from RPL has a 25% chance of having a live birth even without any active treatment.[2]

The definition of RPL differs in different countries. In UK, three or more miscarriages in the first trimester are considered as RPL. The Dutch and American guidelines define RPL as the loss of two or more pregnancies. Causes for RPL are varied. It may be due to luteal phase defect (hormonal) or due to chromosomal problems like balanced translocations. The other suggested causes are anomalies in the uterus like bicornuate or subseptate uterus, immunological causes involving antiphospholipid antibodies, aberrations in the natural killer cells, and thrombophilia.[3]

A pregnancy needs to go through the phases of implantation, embryonic growth, and normal placentation to result in a healthy baby. Heparins are increasingly considered to play an important role in the implantation process and hence are important for management of growth problems of the fetus. There are different schools of thought regarding the management of RPL with heparins. One group has indicated the presence of thrombophilic markers in RPL for starting thromboprophylaxis in RPL patients. Another group has strongly advised against treatment with heparin or aspirin in the absence of a diagnosis of acquired or inherited thrombophilia.[4] There is occurrence of thrombosis in the placenta even if antiphospholipid antibody is present or not in many patients. This indicates the presence of other causes for the fetal loss which has occurred.[5] The main factor which is responsible for a successful pregnancy outcome is actually the tolerance of the immune system to the fetus.

■ HEPARIN

Low molecular weight heparins (LMWHs) have a molecular weight of 4,500–5,000 daltons. Unfractionated heparin (UFH) has a molecular weight of 15,000 daltons. The LMWHs are prepared by depolymerization of unfractionated heparin. LMWHs are preferred over UFH because of the following reasons—more plasma half-life, can be used at lesser doses than UFH, has a response which is more predictable, laboratory monitoring is not essential, known to produce lesser microvascular bleeding than UFH in trials, and there is a lesser risk of thrombocytopenia and osteoporosis.[6]

The tests used for monitoring of therapy are not needed when LMWHs are used. If needed, the levels can be monitored with the Hep test and anti-Xa assay. Anti-Xa assay is available commonly. Monitoring is essential if the patient is obese or has renal insufficiency. It needs to be done 4 hours after a dose. The therapeutic range is 0.6–1 IU/mL. For over dosage, protamine can be used. It can neutralize the antithrombin activity totally but will cause only a partial neutralization of anti-Xa function. It needs to be administered if any procedure needs to be done within 8 hours of the drug being injected. The most common heparin being used at present in many trials is enoxaparin.[7] The other LMWH preparation being tried is tinzaparin sodium. Both enoxaparin and tinzaparin have different properties in their biochemical nature and pharmacological action which may contribute to their different clinical actions.[8] While enoxaparin is prepared by chemical processes, Tinzaparin is prepared by an enzymatic process. This is the reason they show contrasts in the way they exhibit inhibition against factor Xa and factor IIa. Heparins are used alone for the purpose of thromboprophylaxis by some clinicians. Many give an extended treatment by adding steroids, ASA, folic acid, and progesterone preparations along with enoxaparin.[9] The usage of LMWHs is supposed to be beneficial in preventing a pregnancy loss by their anti-inflammatory complement activity and anticoagulant activity.[10,11]

Mode of Action

The action of heparin in antiphospholipid syndrome (APS) is due to its anticoagulation effect.[12] LMWHs can prevent the binding of antiphospholipid antibodies to the trophoblast cells. This will benefit by helping the trophoblastic invasion and differentiation which can be damaged by the antiphospholipid antibodies. Placental apoptosis is prevented by heparins as they can increase Bcl-2 which is an antiapoptotic protein.[10] They protect the placenta from inflammatory injury as they can prevent the activation of complement factors in vitro. Trophoblastic invasiveness is also increased by heparins as they increase matrix metalloproteinases in trophoblastic cells. Heparins directly bind anticardiolipin antibodies and neutralize them. The above actions of heparins are independent of their main action of inhibition of thrombosis and anticoagulant action.

Use of Heparins in Thrombosis

Heparin usage is established in venous thromboembolism and pulmonary embolism. It also has benefits as a thromboprophylactic agent. The usage of heparins in APS is warranted if there is occurrence of RPL which can be unexplained second trimester or third trimester loss, fetal demise, early onset severe preeclampsia, pregnancy-related thrombosis (arterial or venous), severe growth restricted fetus, autoimmune disorders, false positive VDRL testing, prolonged coagulation studies, and positive autoantibody titers.

Use of Heparin in Hereditary Thrombophilia

Many clinicians are using LMWH in their practice for prevention of RPLs.[13] Randomized trials have been done on the association of RPL with hereditary thrombophilia. The answers obtained were not uniform. Different groups have published different results. In the year 2004, a group of French researchers compared a RPL patient group using ASA with a RPL group of patients using heparin as therapy. The randomized trial reported that LMWH was superior to ASA in the management of RPL. A similar study was done by a group from Jordan in 2008. Their results also showed that LMWH was superior to ASA.[14] A different result was reported by a group from Canada who showed that there is no difference in the live birth rates when either LMWH plus ASA are used or aspirin is used alone. This was conducted in 2009 and was termed as the HepASA Trial.[14]

Use of Heparin in Antiphospholipid Syndrome

In patients with RPL and APS, both low-dose aspirin and LMWH in prophylactic doses are given[13] (enoxaparin 1 mg/kg sc once daily). Treatment can be started for both prior embryonic loss and fetal loss. If the patient has prior pregnancy losses and had a thrombotic episode in a previous pregnancy, they need to be maintained on thromboprophylaxis. LMWHs are started in periconceptional period or when the urine pregnancy test is positive. Enoxaparin is given twice daily as a therapeutic dose. If the patient is noncompliant or she finds it to be expensive, warfarin can be given from the second trimester. Warfarin needs to be stopped before delivery and heparin therapy started again. The INR should be monitored during treatment with warfarin. During treatment with prophylactic doses of heparin, factor Xa levels can be monitored.

If there is a history of early preeclampsia in previous pregnancy, low-dose heparin and LMWH can be started in the next pregnancy.

Planning of delivery should be done when a patient is on heparin therapy. Heparin should be stopped 12 hours before delivery and restarted 12 hours after delivery of the baby.

Patients diagnosed with APS should be given thromboprophylaxis with LMWH in the postpartum period for at least 12 weeks. There is a high incidence of thrombosis in the puerperal period. Therapeutic doses of heparin should be given if there were thrombotic events. If RPL or early preeclampsia had occurred, prophylactic heparin should be given. Patients with APS should be ambulated early in the puerperal period and pneumatic compression stockings usage should be encouraged if it is a cesarean delivery.

■ CONCLUSION

Therapy with heparin for women with RPL is considered as safe for the mother and the baby. The incidences of bleeding episodes, thrombotic episodes, and the occurrence of heparin-induced thrombocytopenia are rare. In patients with RPL and APS, treatment with heparin is better than no treatment being offered.

■ REFERENCES

1. Horsager R, Roberts SW, Rogers VL, Santiago-Muñoz PC, Worley KC, Hoffman BL (Eds). Williams Obstetrics, 24th edition. US: McGraw Hill Professional; 2014.
2. Brenner B. Inherited thrombophilia and pregnancy loss. Best Pract Res Clin Haematol. 2003;16:311-20.
3. Saravelos SH, Regan L. Unexplained recurrent pregnancy loss. Obstet Gynecol Clin North Am. 2014;41(1):157-66.
4. de Jong PG, Kaandorp S, Di Nisio M, et al. Aspirin and/or heparin for women with unexplained recurrent miscarriage with or without inherited thrombophilia. Cochrane Database Syst Rev. 2014;7:CD004734.
5. Farquharson RG, Jauniaux E, Exalto N. ESHRE Special Interest Group for Early Pregnancy (SIGEP) Updated and revised nomenclature for description of early pregnancy events. Hum Reprod. 2005;20:3008-11.
6. Hirsh J, Guyatt G, Lewis SZ. Reflecting on eight editions of the American College of Chest Physicians antithrombotic guidelines. Chest. 2008;133(6):1293-5.
7. Duhl AJ, Paidas MJ, Ural SH, et al. Antithrombotic therapy and pregnancy: concensus report and recommendations for prevention and treatment of venous thromboembolism and adverse pregnancy outcomes. Am J Obstet Gynecol. 2007;197:457.e1-457.
8. Fawzy M, Shokeir T, El-Tatongy M, et al. Treatment options and pregnancy outcome in women with idiopathic recurrent miscarriage: a randomized placebo-controlled study. Arch Gynecol Obstet. 2008;278:33-8.
9. Van Horn JT, Craven C, Ward K, et al. Histologic features of placentas and abortion specimens from women with antiphospholipid and antiphospholipid like syndromes. Placenta. 2004;25:642-8.

10. Di Simone N, Ferrazzani S, Castellani R, et al. Heparin and low-dose aspirin restore placental human chorionic gonadotrophin secretion abolished by antiphospholipid antibody-containing sera. Hum Reprod. 1997;12:2061-5.
11. Laskin CA, Spitzer KA, Clark CA, et al. Low molecular weight heparin and aspirin for recurrent pregnancy loss: results from the randomized, controlled HepASA Trial. J Rheumatol. 2009;36(2):279-87.
12. Kutteh WH, Ermel LD. A clinical trial for the treatment of antiphospholipid antibody-associated recurrent pregnancy loss with lower dose heparin and aspirin. Am J Reprod Immunol. 1996;35(4):402-7.
13. Jauniaux E, Farquharson RG, Christiansen OB, et al. Evidence-based guidelines for the investigation and medical treatment of recurrent miscarriage. Human reproduction. 2006;21(9):2216-22.
14. McNamee K, Dawood F, Farquharson R. Recurrent miscarriage and thrombophilia: an update. Curr Opin Obstet Gynecol. 2012;24:229-34.

Chapter 8

Endocrinological Perspectives in Recurrent Pregnancy Loss

Pratik Tambe, Sini S Venugopal

■ BACKGROUND

Conception, implantation and the maintenance of pregnancy requires a synchronized balance among various endocrinological, immunological, genetic, anatomical and environmental factors. Pregnancy losses in human pregnancies are common and approximately 8–15% of all pregnancy losses and recurrent pregnancy losses are postulated to be due to endocrine factors.[1,2] Hence, endocrine abnormalities need to be evaluated in patients with history of recurrent pregnancy loss. Diagnosis and treatment of these endocrine abnormalities can help in improving both maternal and fetal outcomes.

The major endocrinological causes of RPL are:
- Thyroid dysfunction
- Polycystic ovaries
- Obesity
- Hyperinsulinemia and insulin resistance
- Hypersecretion of luteinizing hormone (LH)
- Hyperandrogenemia
- Hyperhomocysteinemia
- Hyperprolactinemia
- Luteal phase deficiency
- Low serum human chorionic gonadotropin (hCG) levels.

■ THYROID DYSFUNCTION

Thyroid disease is one of the most common endocrine abnormalities seen in pregnant women. It affects 2–5% of pregnant women and is associated with adverse pregnancy outcomes.[3,4]

Maternal dietary iodine deficiency results in impaired maternal and fetal thyroid hormone synthesis. Low thyroid hormone values stimulate increased pituitary thyroid-stimulating hormone (TSH) production and the increased TSH stimulates thyroid growth, resulting in maternal and fetal goiter. In areas of severe iodine deficiency, thyroid nodules can be present in as many as 30% of pregnant women. Severe iodine deficiency in pregnant women has been associated with increased rates of pregnancy loss, stillbirth, and increased perinatal and infant mortality.

Normal levels of thyroid hormone are essential for neuronal migration, myelination, and other structural changes of the fetal brain. Because thyroid hormones are needed throughout pregnancy, iodine deficiency affects both maternal and fetal thyroid hormone production, and insufficient iodine intake can lead to detrimental effects. Specifically, maternal and fetal iodine deficiency in pregnancy have adverse effects on the cognitive function of offspring.

Children whose mothers were severely iodine deficient during pregnancy may exhibit cretinism, characterized by profound intellectual impairment, deaf-mutism, and motor rigidity. Iodine deficiency is known to be the leading cause of preventable intellectual deficits worldwide.

The recommended upper thyroid-stimulating hormone (TSH) value in the first trimester in both the 2011 and 2012 American Thyroid Association (ATA) guidelines is 2.50 mIU/L and 3.00 mIU/L in the second and the third trimester.[5,6]

The latest 2017 ATA Thyroid and Pregnancy Guidelines recommend that an upper reference limit (URL) of 4.0 mIU/L can be used if internal or transferable pregnancy-specific reference ranges of TSH are not available.[5]

As regards the incidence of thyroglobulin antibody (TgAb) and thyroid peroxidase antibody (TPOAb) in patients with recurrent losses, some studies report a higher incidence while others demonstrated no difference when compared to healthy controls. A meta-analysis of eight studies that included 460 antibody-positive patients and 1,923 controls noted a significant association between thyroid antibody positivity and recurrent pregnancy loss (OR 2.3; 95% CI 1.5–3.5).[3]

Hence, the data for an association between thyroid antibodies and RPL is less robust than for sporadic loss. This finding may be because RPL has many potential causes, and endocrine dysfunction may only account for 15–20% of all such cases. Some studies have reported that women with RPL who were antithyroid antibody positive also demonstrated higher levels of anticardiolipin antibody and other nonorgan-specific antibodies.

Overt Hypothyroidism

Maternal hypothyroidism is the most frequent endocrine disorder as well as thyroid disorder in pregnancy which is associated with a number of adverse pregnancy complications as well as detrimental fetal effects.[7-10]

Treatment with levothyroxine is indicated to prevent the adverse complications and improve the pregnancy outcome.[5,11,12]

Subclinical Hypothyroidism

Subclinical hypothyroidism (SCH) is defined as an elevated TSH concentration with concurrent normal thyroid hormone concentrations. It is estimated to affect up to 2–3% of all pregnancies as per the latest 2017 ATA guidelines.[7]

Subclinical hypothyroidism may not have any overt manifestations, but it is a disease which heralds the onset of pathophysiological changes and metabolic aberrations of overt hypothyroidism.[13] Thyroid hormones play a vital role in maintaining normal Na^+/K^+ ATPase (the sodium pump) activity. T3 and T4 increase the expression of sodium pump in the plasma membrane of cells.[14] This sodium pump is essential for maintaining the normal membrane potential and it has more significance for excitable cells like nerve cells, which depend on this pump to respond to stimuli and transmission of impulses.

Hypothyroidism is associated with hypercholesterolemia and dyslipidemia. Thyroid hormones stimulate cholesterol synthesis by inducing HMG-CoA reductase which leads to the increased intracellular cholesterol seen in hyperthyroidism. In hypothyroid patients, in spite of reduced HMG-CoA reductase activity, there is increase in total cholesterol, mainly due to increased level of low density lipoprotein (LDL) and intermediate density lipoprotein (IDL) cholesterol. In hypothyroidism, there is a 60% increase in the plasma cholesterol level with a 22% reduction in erythrocyte membrane cholesterol content.[15] This membrane cholesterol plays a crucial role in the regulation of sodium pump activity.

Levothyroxine treatment in women with RPL and SCH is as yet controversial. A reduced risk of pregnancy loss was seen with levothyroxine treatment in a retrospective analysis of 5,405 pregnant women with SCH.[16,17] But, levothyroxine therapy during pregnancy has its own limitations owing to its adverse fetal neurodevelopment effects.[18] Hence, the benefits of treatment need to be weighed against the risks.

The European Thyroid Association Guidelines for the management of SCH in pregnancy and in children state that SCH arising before conception or during gestation should be treated with levothyroxine. The ATA also recommends levothyroxine treatment for pregnant women with SCH (with TSH above trimester specific ranges) and TPO-Ab, or SCH (with TSH above 10 mIU/L).

Hyperthyroidism

The prevalence of overt hyperthyroidism in pregnancy is about 0.2–0.4% and that of subclinical hyperthyroidism in pregnancy is about 1.7–2%. Overt hyperthyroidism (most commonly caused by Graves' disease) is associated with higher frequency of pregnancy complications.[5] According to the Endocrine Society Clinical Practice Guideline (ESCPG) and the ATA, hyperthyroidism needs to be treated with antithyroid drugs propylthiouracil (PTU) or methimazole (MMI).

Thyroid Autoimmunity

This is defined as the presence of thyroid antibodies against thyroid peroxidase (TPO-Ab) and/or thyroglobulin (Tg-Ab) in combination with a normal or abnormal thyroid function. It has an incidence of 8–14% among women of reproductive age group.[19,20] The most frequent cause of hypothyroidism in women of reproductive age group is autoimmune thyroid disease. TPO-Ab is one of the markers of RPL and predisposes to hypothyroidism, but the majority of women having TPO-Ab are euthyroid. Greater risk of miscarriage associated with thyroid autoimmunity could be due to the increased autoimmune imbalance that leads to a greater rejection of the fetal graft.[21]

It is recommended to perform thyroid screening (TSH and TPO-Ab) in women with RPL. If women with TPO-Ab and RPL are pregnant, check for TSH levels and hypothyroidism, if present, should be treated with levothyroxine **(Flowchart 1)**.[5] But, if patient is euthyroid, then levothyroxine treatment to improve the pregnancy outcomes is still controversial.

Flowchart 1: Testing for thyroid dysfunction in pregnancy.

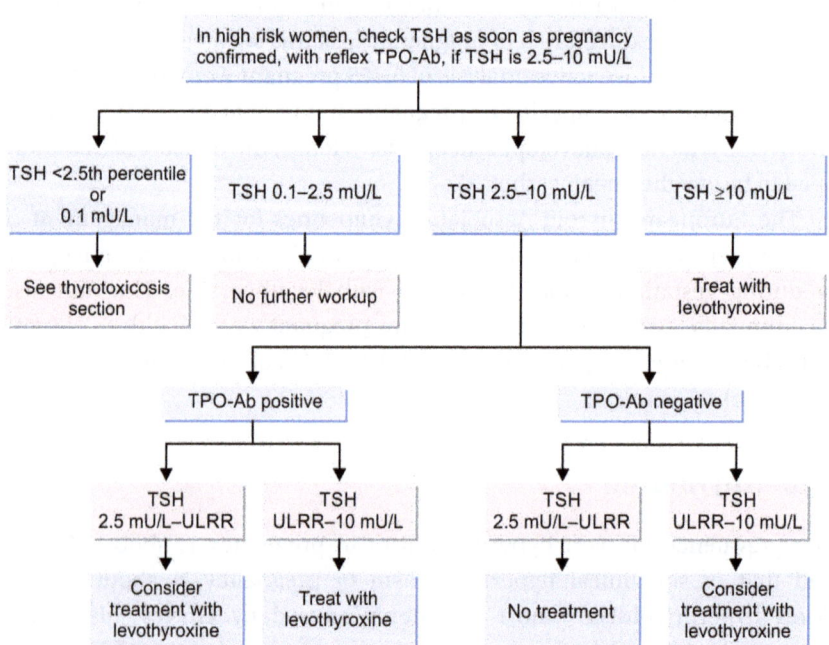

(TPO: thyroid peroxidase; TSH: thyroid-stimulating hormone; ULRR: upper limit of the reference range)

POLYCYSTIC OVARY SYNDROME

Polycystic ovary syndrome (PCOS) is the most common cause of anovulatory infertility and a common abnormality among women with RPL. Spontaneous and recurrent pregnancy loss occurs in 40% of women with PCOS[22] mainly due to the various metabolic associations of PCOS.[23,24]

OBESITY

Obesity has various detrimental effects on the female reproductive function through hyperinsulinemia and hyperandrogenemia.[25,26] Maternal obesity with BMI >30 kg/m^2 has been reported as an independent risk factor for euploid miscarriage.[27] Insulin resistance is the main linking factor among obesity, PCOS, and RPL.[28] Obesity is associated with a reduction in progesterone (a potent anti-inflammatory agent) by corpus luteum thereby reduced decidualization.[29-31] Another study reported an alteration in endometrial haptoglobin, compared with lean counterparts.[32,33] Deregulation of leptin levels has been correlated with pathogenesis of RPL.[34]

HYPERINSULINEMIA AND INSULIN RESISTANCE

Insulin resistance (IR) is an independent risk factor for early pregnancy loss in women with or without PCOS. IR and subsequent hyperinsulinemia is the common linking factor in the pathophysiology of miscarriage in PCOS.[35,36] Different mechanisms by which it causes RPL include its effect on oocyte maturation, glucose uptake and metabolism, implantation, altered expression of *HOXA10* gene, reduction of serum glycodelin (inhibits endometrial immune response), and insulin-like growth factor binding protein-1 (IGFBP-1) (facilitates embryo adhesion) concentration.[37,38] Impaired glucose uptake caused by downregulation of IGF-1 results in blastocyst apoptosis.

Hyperinsulinemia may increase the level of PAI-1 which induces a hypofibrinolytic state and villous thrombosis leading to trophoblastic hypoplasia and miscarriage.[39] Hyperinsulinemia and IR cause excessive glucose transport to the fetal environment by cytotrophoblasts (by upregulation of the GLUT-1 glucose transporter system), leading to miscarriage.

HYPERSECRETION OF LUTEINIZING HORMONE

Hypersecretion of LH is a common finding in PCOS. High serum concentration of LH with or without PCOS, have been associated with an increased prevalence of pregnancy loss.[2] Raised follicular LH causes premature oocyte aging and poor endometrial development.[36]

■ HYPERANDROGENEMIA

Elevated androgen levels (testosterone and androstenedione) have been found to play a role in miscarriage/RPL with or without PCOS in some studies but other studies have found conflicting reports.[35]

Sex steroids regulate uterine receptivity for embryo implantation by controlling the expression of the *HOXA10* gene. Elevated testosterone in PCOS downregulates the expression of *HOXA10* gene, thereby decreasing the uterine receptivity and implantation. Free testosterone or free androgen index (FAI) are the most sensitive methods of determining hyperandrogenemia. Women with elevated androgens have reduced concentration of expression of the endometrial protein PP14 (glycodelin A) in the periimplantation period and also have poor oocyte quality.

■ HYPERHOMOCYSTEINEMIA

Hyperhomocysteinemia is a risk factor for venous thromboembolism and is associated with adverse pregnancy outcomes including neural tube defects, pre-eclampsia, placental abruption, and RPL.

In a meta-analysis of case-control studies, an association was found between RPL and fasting plasma homocysteine.[40,41] Recent studies have reported conflicting results.[42,43] Hyperhomocysteinemia has been suggested as a linking factor between PCOS and RPL.[23,39] RPL affected PCOS patients seemed to have an increased incidence of hyperhomocysteinemia compared to women with RPL but without PCOS. The thrombogenic milieu due to hyperhomocysteinemia results in microthrombi formation in the placental bed leading to poor placentation.

Various studies have reported the role of folic acid, vitamin B_6, vitamin B_{12}, and low molecular weight heparin (LMWH) in improving the pregnancy outcomes in women with hyperhomocysteinemia.

■ HYPERPROLACTINEMIA

Hyperprolactinemia is associated with miscarriage, especially in women who have experienced unexplained RPL.[44,45]

Prolactin levels are usually evaluated more for ovulatory dysfunction than for RPL. However, hyperprolactinemia if found associated with RPL can be considered for treatment.

■ LUTEAL PHASE DEFICIENCY

Luteal phase deficiency (LPD) is a condition wherein there is insufficient progesterone exposure to maintain a regular secretory endometrium and to allow for normal embryo implantation and growth.[46] LPD can be caused by several endocrinopathies, including stress, PCOS, and prolactin disorders.[1,47] Studies have failed to confirm a strong association between LPD and RPL. LPD testing is not routinely recommended in women with RPL, though reduced levels of progesterone are found in women with RPL.

Progesterone production triggers favorable morphological and physiological changes in the endometrium creating a suitable environment for the embryo during the implantation window.[48] Studies on animals and humans suggest that progesterone maintains pregnancy by downregulation of Th1 cytokines and stimulation of Th2 cytokines.

While the PROMISE Trial showed that progesterone therapy in the first trimester of pregnancy did not result in a significantly higher rate of live births among women with a history of unexplained recurrent miscarriages (65.8% vs. 63.3%),[49] there has been criticism of the trial regarding the dosage of progesterone therapy used during the trial.

The most recent Cochrane meta-analysis published October 2018 considered 13 trials with 2,556 women. The authors concluded that progesterone supplementation probably reduces the number of miscarriages compared to placebo (RR 0.69). There is a slight benefit as regards improved live birth rate (RR 1.11), reduction of preterm births (RR 0.59), and a possible reduction in stillbirths (RR 0.38).[50]

■ DIABETES MELLITUS

Evaluation for diabetes is advised with clinical suspicion. The glycosylated hemoglobin test is adequate as a screening test.[51] The best investigation is the oral glucose tolerance test (OGTT), but it is the most expensive and is inconvenient. Fasting plasma glucose would miss people with impaired glucose tolerance. Glycosylated hemoglobin does not require fasting, and may be the best compromise.[52] A two hour single step, single value with a cut off of >140 mg/dL has been proposed by WHO and is endorsed by many international organizations including the Diabetes in India Study Group (DIPSI).

■ LOW SERUM hCG LEVELS

Women with low or suboptimally increasing serum human chorionic gonadotropin (hCG) levels are at much higher risk of miscarriage. These are commonly measured in ART pregnancies and it may be worthwhile to have serial estimations in patients with recurrent losses though there is insufficient guidance regarding adopting this as a routine practice.

CONCLUSION

Endocrine dysfunction is one of the important factors responsible for recurrent pregnancy loss. An altered endocrine profile results especially in early pregnancy losses. The associations with thyroid disorders, PCOS, obesity, hyperinsulinemia and other frequently occurring endocrine issues have been dealt with.

Currently, there is no strong evidence to support routine testing of LH, androgens, homocysteine or prolactin in RPL. Similarly, there is no evidence to support routine metformin therapy for IR with RPL.

Future developments in diagnostic testing and evidence of efficacy of treatment of endocrine disorders among patients with RPL are much awaited, for the ultimate goal of any clinician is not just to aim at successful implantation but a successful pregnancy outcome.

REFERENCES

1. Ke RW. Endocrine basis for RL. Obstet Gynaecol Clin North Am. 2014;41:103-12.
2. Roy S, Dasgupta A. The effects of altered membrane cholesterol levels on sodium pump activity in subclinical hypothyroidism. Endocrinol Metab (Seoul). 2017;32(1):129-39.
3. van den Boogard, Vissenberg R, Land JA, et al. Significance of (sub)clinical thyroid dysfunction and thyroid autoimmunity before conception and in early pregnancy: a systematic review. Hum Reprod Update. 2011;17(5):605-19.
4. Vissenberg R, Manders VD, Mastenbroek S, et al. Pathophysiological aspects of thyroid hormone disorders/thyroid peroxidase auto-antibody and reproduction. Hum Reprod Update. 2015;21(3):378-87.
5. Alexander EK, Pearce EN, Brent GA, et al. Guidelines of the American Thyroid Association for the diagnosis and Management of Thyroid disease during pregnancy and the postpartum. Thyroid. 2017;27(3):315-89.
6. Taylor PN, Minassian C, Rehman A, et al. TSH levels and risk of miscarriage in women on long term levothyroxine: a community based study. J Clin Endocrinol Metab. 2014;99(10):3895-902.
7. Lazarus JH, Bestwick JP, Channon S, et al. Antenatal thyroid screening and childhood cognitive function. New Engl J Med. 2012;366(6):493-501.
8. Hirsch D, Levy S, Nadler V, et al. Pregnancy outcomes in women in severe hypothyroidism. Europian J Endocrinol. 2013;169:313-20.
9. Chan S, Boelaert K. Optimal management of hypothyroidism, hypothyroxinaemia and euthyroid thyroid peroxidase antibody positivity in preconception and in pregnancy. Clin Endocrinol (Oxf). 2015;82(3):313-26.
10. Vaidya B, Hubalewska-Dydejczyk A, Laurberg P, et al. Treatment and screening of hypothyroidism in pregnancy: results of a European Survey. Eur J Endocrinol. 2012;166:49-54.
11. El Baba KA, Azar ST. Thyroid dysfunction in pregnancy. Int J Gen Med. 2012;5:227-30.

12. Lazarus J, Brown RS, Daumerie C, et al. European thyroid association guidelines for the management of sunclinical hypothyroidism in pregnancy and in children. Eur Thyroid J. 2014;3:76-94.
13. Koromilas C, Liapi C, Zarros A, et al. Inhibition of Na(+), K(+) - ATPase in the hypothalamus, pons and cerebellum of the offspring rat due to experimentally induced material hypothyroidism. J Matern Fetal Neonatal Med. 2015;28:1438-44.
14. Lambropaulos N, Garcia A, Clarke RJ. Stimulation of Na(+), K (+) - ATPase activity as a possible driving force in cholesterol evolution. J Membr Biol. 2016:249:251-9.
15. Karbownik-Lowinska M, Marcinkowska M, Stepniak J, et al. TSH >= 2.5 mIU/l is associated with the increased oxidative damage to membrane lipids in women of child bearing age with normal thyroid tests. Horm Metab Res. 2017;49(5):321-6.
16. Maraka S, Mwangi R, McCoy RG, et al. Thyroid hormone treatment among pregnant women with subclinical hypothyroidism: US national assessment. BMJ. 2017;356:i6865.
17. Lepoutre T, Debieve F, Gruson D, et al. Reduction of miscarriage through universal screening and treatment of thyroid autoimmune diseases. Gynecol Obstet. 2012;74:256-73.
18. Korevaar TI, Muetzel R, Medici M, et al. Association of maternal thyroid function during early pregnancy with offspring IQ and brain morphology in childhood: a population-based prospective cohort study. Lancet Diabetes Endocrinol. 2016;7(8):629-37.
19. Lata K, Dutta P, Sridhar S, et al. Thyroid autoimmunity and obstetric outcomes in women in recurrent miscarriage. A case–control study. Endocr Connect. 2013;2(2):118-24.
20. Mannisto T, Mendola P, Grewal J, et al. Thyroid diseases: contemporary US cohort. J Clin Endocrinol Metab. 2013;98:2725-33.
21. Yan J, Sripada S, Saravelos SH, et al. Thyroid peroxidase antibody in women in unexplained recurrent miscarriage: prevalence, prognostic value and response to thyroxine therapy. Fertil Steril. 2012;98:378-82.
22. Liu L, Tong X, Jiang L, et al. A comparison of the miscarriage rate between women with and without polycystic ovary syndrome undergoing IVF treatment. Eur J Obstet Gynecol Reprod Biol. 2014;176:178-82.
23. Chakraborty P, Goswami SK, Rajani S, et al. Recurrent pregnancy loss in polycystic ovary syndrome: role of hyperhomocysteinemia and insulin resistance. PLoS One. 2013;8(5):64446.
24. Ashaq L, Al Mazer Y, Al Qahtani N. Recurrent pregnancy loss in patients in polycystic syndrome: a case control study. Open J Obstet Gynaecol. 2017;7:1073-85.
25. Sugiura-Ogasawara M. Recurrent pregnancy loss and density. Best Pract Res Clin Obstet Gynaecol. 2015;29(4):489-97.
26. Cavalcante MB, Samo M, Peixoto AB, et al. Obesity and recurrent miscarriage: a systematic review and meta-analysis. J Obstet Gynaecol Res. 2018;13799.
27. Catalano PM, Shankar K. Obesity and pregnancy: mechanism of short term and long term adverse consequences for mother and child. BMJ. 2017;356.
28. Boots CE, Bernardi LA, Stephenson MD. Frequency of recurrent miscarriage is increased in obese women in recurrent early pregnancy loss. Fertil Steril. 2014;102(2):455-9.

29. Tremellen K, Syedi N, Tan S, et al. Metabolic endotoxaemia- a potential novel link between ovarian inflammation and impaired progesterone production. Gynecol Endocrinol. 2015;31(4):309-12.
30. Goh JY, He S, Allen JC, et al. Maternal obesity is associated with a low serum progesterone level in early pregnancy. Horm Mol Biol Clin Investig. 2016;27(3):97-100.
31. Rhee JS, Saben JL, Mayes AL, et al. Diet induced obesity impairs endometrial stromal cell decidualization a potential role for impaired autophagy. Hum Reprod. 2016;31:1315-26.
32. Metwelly M, Preece R, Thomas J, et al. A proteomic analysis of the endometrium in obese and overweight women in recurrent miscarriage: preliminary evidence for an endometrium defect. Reprod Biol Endocrinol. 2015;12:75.
33. Agarwal A, Aponte-Mellado A, Premkumar BJ, et al. The effects of oxidative stress on female reproduction: a review. Reprod Biol Endocrinol. 2012;10:49.
34. Pérez-Pérez A, Toro A, Vilariño-García T, et al. Leptin action in normal and pathological pregnancies. J Cell Mol Med. 2018;22(2):716-27.
35. Ispasoiu CA, Chicea R, Stamatian FV, et al. High fasting insulin levels and insulin resistance may be linked to idiopathic recurrent pregnancy loss: a case-control study. Int J Endocrinol. 2013;2013:576926.
36. Shanmugham D, Vidhyalakhhmi RK, Shivamusthy HM. The effect of baseline serum LH (Leutenizing Hormone) levels on follicular development, ovulation, conception and pregnancy outcome in infertile patients in polycystic ovary syndrome. Int J Reprod Contracept Obstet Gynaecol. 2018;7(1):318-22.
37. Wani AA, Gul I, Jabeen F, et al. Relationship of insulin resistance in recurrent pregnancy loss. Int J Reprod Contracept Obstet Gynaecol. 2017;6(4):1312-7.
38. Tamara T, Elk holy A, Elsaed N, et al. Association between unexplained recurrent miscarriage and insulin resistance. Int J Reprod Med Gynecol. 2018;4(1):001-5.
39. Kazeroni T, Ghaffarpasand F, Asadi N, et al. Correlation between thrombophilia and recurrent pregnancy loss in patients with polycystic ovary syndrome: A comparative study. J Chin Med Assoc. 2013;76:282-8.
40. Puri M, Kaur L, Walia GK, et al. MTHFR C677T polymorphism, folate, vitamin B12 and homocysteine in recurrent pregnancy loss: a case control study among North Indian Woman. J. Perinat Med. 2013;41:549-54.
41. Mukhopadhyay I, Pruthviraj V, Rao PS, et al. Hyperhomocysteinemia in recurrent pregnancy loss and the effect of folic acid and vitamin B12 on homocysteine levels: a prospective analysis. J Reprod Contracept Obstet Gynaecol. 2017;6(6):2258-61.
42. Creus M, Deulofeu R, Penarrubia J, et al. Plasma homocysteine and vitamin B12 serum levels red blood cell folate concentration, C677T MTHFR reductase gene mutation and risk of recurrent miscarriage: a case control study in Spain. Clin Chem Lab Med. 2013;51:693-9.
43. Lee GS, Park JC, Rhee JH, et al. Etiologic characteristic and index pregnancy outcomes of recurrent pregnancy loss in Korean women. Obstet Gynaecol Sci. 2016;59:379-87.
44. Li W, Ma N, Laird SM, et al. The relationship between serum prolactin concentration and pregnancy outcome in women in unexplained recurrent miscarriage. J Obstet Gynaecol. 2013;33:285-8.

45. Triggianese P, Perricone C, Perricone R, et al. Prolactin and natural killer cells: evaluating the neuro-endocrine immune axis in women with primary infertility and recurrent spontaneous abortion. Am J Reprod Immunol. 2015;73:56-65.
46. Palomba S, Santagni S, La Sala GB. Progesterone administration for luteal phase deficiency in human reproduction: an old or new issue. J Ovarian Res. 2015;8:77.
47. Shah D, Nagarajan N. Luteal deficiency in first trimester. Indian J Endocrinol Metab. 2013;17(1):44-9.
48. Dante G, Vaccaro V, Facchinetti F. Use of progestagens during early pregnancy. Facts Views Vis Obgy. 2013;5(1):66-71.
49. Coomarasamy A, Williams H, Truchanowicz E, et al. A randomized trial of progesterone in women with recurrent miscarriages (PROMISE). N Engl J Med. 2015;373:2141-8.
50. Haas DM, Hathaway TJ, Ramsey PS. Progestogen for preventing miscarriage in women with recurrent miscarriage of unclear etiology. Cochrane Database Syst Rev. 2018;(10):CD003511.
51. Jeve B, Davies W. Evidence-based management of recurrent miscarriages. J Hum Reprod Sci. 2014;7(3):159-9.
52. Malkani S, DeSilva T. Controversies on how diabetes is diagnosed. Curr Opin Endocrinol Diabetes Obes. 2012;19:97-103.

Chapter 9

Cervical Factors in Recurrent Pregnancy Loss

Alpesh Gandhi, Kirtan M Vyas

■ INTRODUCTION

Human reproduction is a complex process. It has been found in different studies that approximately 15–30% of fertilized ova fail to get converted into a viable pregnancy. Kutteh WH et al. in 1995 reported an incidence of around 25% for preclinical loss of pregnancy and a clinical miscarriage rate of around 13%. Although majority of the miscarriages are a result of an abnormal fetus, other causes for pregnancy loss are also significant. In almost 70% first trimester losses and 30% of second trimester losses, the fetus is found to be normal. Recurrent pregnancy loss (RPL) is a major setback to the couple eager to become parents and a challenge to the clinicians. Advances in genetics in conjunction with advances in the knowledge of physiology and immunology have helped clinicians to achieve some promising results in the management of this condition. It is also worth noting that improvement in imaging techniques, hormonal studies, advanced endoscopic procedures, and drugs have all contributed to achieve successful management of recurrent pregnancy loss. The rate of recurrence after a single miscarriage is less than 30% and 80–90% of women will have a successful pregnancy after a spontaneous abortion.

Recurrent pregnancy loss is two or more consecutive spontaneous losses before 20 weeks of gestation or a fetus weighing less than 500 g. Overall incidence of RPL is 0.5–1%.[1] Causes of RPL can be genetic, anatomic, endocrine, immunologic, infectious, environmental, and often an overlapping of all these. In almost 50% of patients of RPL, no definite cause can be identified.

■ CONTRIBUTORY CERVICAL FACTORS

Structural and functional abnormalities in female genital tract are an important cause of RPL. An incompetent cervix is a major contributory factor for second trimester pregnancy loss. Cervical incompetence is defined as passive painless dilatation of the cervix from second trimester onward resulting in membrane bulging and abortion.[2] Principal structural component in cervix are smooth muscles, collagen, and connective tissue which is the ground substance. In this ground substance, important constituents of the cervix, the glycosaminoglycan—hyaluronic acid, is present. The smooth muscles content is around 30-60%. Cervical changes that occur in women with incompetent cervix are identical to those in parturition, i.e. increased synthesis of collagenases, increased production of hyaluronic acid, and infiltration by inflammatory cells that leads to collagen breakdown, increased water content, and inflammatory cytokines.

■ ETIOPATHOGENESIS

Cervical incompetence may be anatomic or functional. There are many factors which result in cervical incompetence. These include congenital weakness of the internal os sphincter mechanism or cervical incompetence following trauma. Many procedures that lead to cervical trauma include mechanical cervical dilatation for induced abortions, conization, cervical amputation (Fothergill Repair), laceration after a difficult instrumental assisted vaginal delivery, delivery of after coming head in breech presentation or any intrauterine manipulation. In some cases, cervix may be congenitally abnormal as in Müllerian fusion anomalies or exposure to diethylstilbestrol (DES) in utero.[3]

■ DIAGNOSIS

Cervical insufficiency may occur in nulliparous or multiparous women. Congenital causes, surgical dilatation prior to curettage, conization or loop electrosurgical excision procedure (LEEP) may result in cervical incompetence during the first pregnancy itself, while obstetric trauma mostly affects multiparous women. Cervical incompetence due to primary cervical disease is a recurrent problem but when it is secondary to early preterm labor, it is not necessarily recurrent. Cervical insufficiency may be more common amongst obese women, although not supported by literature.

Buckingham has divided cervical incompetence into three different categories:
Category I: Patients with mechanical disruption of fibrous ring due to trauma
Category II: Patients with histological deficit
Category III: Patients having dysfunctional cervical incompetence with no structural or histological defects is due to premature triggering of normal mechanism of cervical dilatation and effacement.

Cervical incompetence can be suspected by history and examination. Majority of patients with cervical insufficiency may be asymptomatic. However some may complain of pelvic pressure, cramping, back pain or increased vaginal discharge. Digital examination is often informative but it is subjective. Digital examination can lead to stimulation of premature uterine contractions, introduction of infection in women with preterm premature rupture of the membranes (PPROM), and antepartum hemorrhage in patients with abnormal placentation.

Ultrasonography can be a very helpful tool to obtain information of cervical incompetence, particularly in women in whom PV examination is not recommended. Transvaginal sonography (TVS) is superior to transabdominal sonography (TAS) for diagnosis of cervical incompetence. TVS is objective and noninvasive so it has an advantage of safety even during pregnancy. It is useful for screening and early detection of changes in supravaginal portion of the cervix and the internal os which are not amenable to PV examination. Shortening of the cervical length, dilatation of the internal os, funneling of the cervix or prolapse of membranes into cervix are signs that suggest cervical incompetence. Henceforth a cervical length which is less than 25 mm between 14 weeks and 26 weeks gestation, dilatation of internal os more than 5 mm before 30 weeks of gestation, and funneling and prolapse of membranes into cervix with shortening of functional cervical length are important criteria to look for when we are evaluating a case of cervical incompetence. But these factors alone do not conclude the diagnosis. A patient has to suffer a clinical pregnancy loss before a final diagnosis is confirmed. In any given case, depending upon severity of the findings, monitoring should be recommended weekly or every 15 days. TVS is helpful to curb the indications of encerclage in cases for which the situation is uncertain. Studies have also demonstrated utility of fetal fibronectin (fFN) testing in addition to cervical length assessment with a significant improvement in prediction of preterm delivery in women with a positive fFN and a cervical length of less than 30 mm.[4]

Cervical incompetence—examination[5]
Interconceptional period:
- Bimanual examination—speculum inspection reveals bilateral or unilateral cervical tear or gaping of cervix up to internal os.

During pregnancy:
- Cervix ≥2 cm dilated and ≥80% effaced with herniating bag of waters through cervix.

Cervical incompetence—evaluation
Interconceptional period:
- Passage of Hegar dilator no. 6 to 8 without resistance beyond internal os and absence of internal os snap on dilators withdrawal, especially in premenstrual time.
- Premenstrual HSG—funnel-shaped shadow. The internal os is supposed to be tight during this time because of effect of progesterone (during proliferative phase even a competent cervix may give a funnel shadow).

During pregnancy:
- Cervical length <2.5 cm in TVS, funneling of upper cervix and width of internal os >5 mm before 14-16 weeks with or without bulging of membrane.[6]

MANAGEMENT

The American College of Obstetricians and Gynecologists (ACOG) in 2014 outlined cervical cerclage as a mainstem treatment for cervical insufficiency. In this procedure, a stitch is placed at the cervicovaginal junction which can benefit women with a history of cervical insufficiency or previous midtrimester loss. It is reasonable to perform cervical cerclage in certain situations:
- Prior midtrimester loss with painless cervical dilatation.
- Prior cerclage for cervical insufficiency.
- History of spontaneous preterm birth (prior to 34 weeks gestation) and a short cervical length (<25 mm) prior to 24 weeks gestation.
- Painless cervical dilatation on physical examination in second trimester.

PRINCIPAL OF CERVICAL ENCERCLAGE

A nonabsorbable encircling suture is placed around the cervix at the level of internal os. It acts by interfering with uterine polarity, preventing internal os and adjacent lower segment from being "taken up". In a proven case of cervical incompetence, it is done around 14-16 weeks or at least 2 weeks earlier than the lowest period of previous wastage, as early as 10th week.

Cervical cerclage is not recommended in patients with short cervix but not having a history of preterm delivery according to ACOG. It is also not practiced routinely for multiple pregnancies with a short cervix as this has been associated with an increased risk for preterm birth. Bed rest is also not found to be effective to treat cervical insufficiency.

As per the Cochrane database, the use of a cervical stitch should not be offered to women at low or medium risk of mid-trimester loss, regardless of cervical length by ultrasound. The role of cervical cerclage for women who have short cervix on ultrasound remains uncertain as the number of randomized women are too few to draw firm conclusions. Cervical cerclage reduces the risk of preterm birth in women at high-risk of preterm birth and probably reduces risk of perinatal deaths. There was no evidence of any differential effect of cerclage based on previous obstetric history or short cervix indications, but data were limited for all clinical groups. The question of whether cerclage is more or less effective than other preventative treatments, particularly vaginal progesterone, remains unanswered.

■ PREOPERATIVE CARE FOR SURGICAL PROCEDURE

- Nil by mouth for 6–8 hours
- Monitoring of anticoagulants and antidiabetics
- Preoperative blood and urine profiles
- Physician fitness.

■ METHODS OF CERVICAL CERCLAGE[7]

It can be performed either transvaginally or transabdominally. Before preparing a patient for this procedure, fetal ultrasound should be performed to confirm viability, gestational age, and to rule out gross congenital anomaly. Any form of active bleeding, PPROM or preterm labor should be excluded. A patient should be explained beforehand regarding possible complications of the procedure including suture displacement, artificial rupture of membranes, and chorioamnionitis.

McDonald Operation (Fig. 1)[7]

It is simple and easy to perform. It consists of a purse-string suture in cervix. The suture material used is a nonabsorbable one, usually prolene, as high as possible into vaginal fornices.

Shirodkar Operation (Fig. 2)[7]

This includes incisions into cervical mucosa anterior and posterior after separating bladder and rectum, respectively. In this procedure, vaginal mucosa is sutured over cerclage suture, which requires delivery by cesarean section. To make the procedure simpler from this original one, incision of

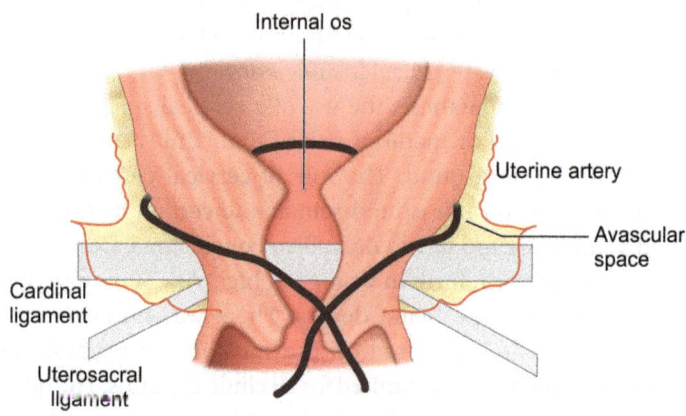

Fig. 1: McDonald operation.[7]

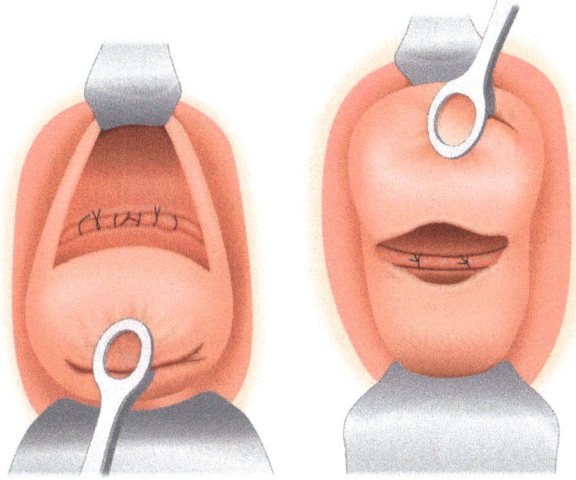

Fig. 2: Shirodkar operation.[7]

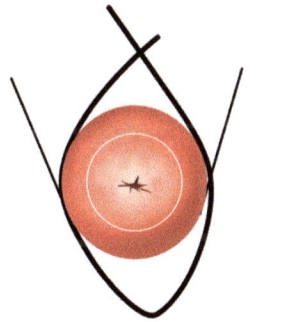

Fig. 3: Espinosa-Flores operation.[8]

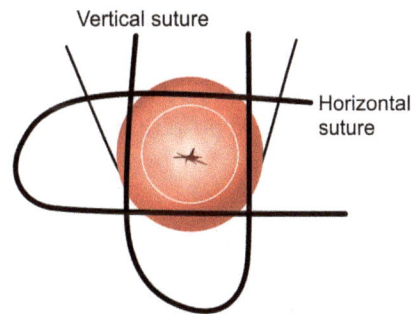

Fig. 4: Wurm operation.[9]

only anterior cervical mucosa is done and it is concluded by tying the suture over intact vaginal mucosa.

Espinosa-Flores Operation (Fig. 3)[8]

It is an emergency procedure popular as rescue cerclage. Two bites are taken into the cervix at 9'o clock and 3'o clock position. One may require displacing herniated bow inside uterus with a Foleys catheter. The suture may be tied over anterior or posterior aspects of the cervix.

Wurm Operation (Fig. 4)[9]

It is a "U" stitch with prolene, one vertically and other horizontally. First suture is a mattress suture placed vertically from 12'o clock to 6'o clock and back to 12'o clock. Suture two is a similar one placed horizontally from 3'o clock to 9'o clock and back to 3'o clock.

POSTOPERATIVE CARE/CONCERNS

- Monitor the patient for fever, chills, nausea, and cramps in abdomen.
- Patient is asked to report if she feels something is bulging out into vagina or leaking per vaginum.
- Postoperative progesterone is continued for next 48 hours for uterine relaxation.
- Antenatal corticosteroids are advised in all these patients for fetal lung maturity at 26–28 weeks.

INDICATIONS OF ABDOMINAL CERCLAGE[10]

- Patients with RPL following extensive cervical conization or amputation.
- Failed vaginal cerclage.
- Mahran in 1978 described abdominal cerclage. The procedure is usually done between 16 and 18 weeks of pregnancy. The suture material is introduced from posterior to anterior aspect of broad ligament close to cervix and inserted again in opposite side from anterior to posterior. The ends are tied posteriorly, to be removed by a posterior colpotomy when required.

CONCLUSION

Cervical factors are one of the important contributory factors for recurrent pregnancy loss. A full examination protocol should be implemented following two or more consecutive losses apart from speculum examination and TVS. Thorough follow-up with cervical encerclage play an important role in management strategies. Regardless of the care, psychological support helps gain confidence of the couple.[5]

REFERENCES

1. Goldenberg RL, Culhane JF, Iams JD, et al. Epidemiology and causes of preterm birth. Lancet. 2008;371(9606):75-84.
2. Fernando A, Daftary SN, Bhide AG. Practical Guide to High Risk Pregnancy and Delivery, 3rd edition, 2008. pp. 262-76.
3. Rackow BW, Arici A. Reproductive performance of women with müllerian anomalies. Curr Opin Obstet Gynecol. 2007;19(3):229-37.
4. Schmitz T, Maillard F, Bessard-Bacquaert S, et al. Selective use of fetal fibronectin detection after cervical length measurement to predict spontaneous preterm delivery in women with preterm labor. Am J Obstet Gynecol. 2006;194(1):138-43.

5. American College of Obstetricians and Gynecologists. Practice Bulletin No. 142: Cerclage for the management of cervical insufficiency. Obstet Gynecol. 2014;123:372-9.
6. Berghella V, Ludmir J, Simonazzi G, et al. Transvaginal cervical cerclage: evidence for perioperative management strategies. Am J Obstet Gynecol. 2013;209(3): 181-92.
7. Berghella V, Baxter JK, Hendrix NW. Cervical assessment by ultrasound for preventing preterm delivery. Cochrane Database Syst Rev. 2013;1:CD007235.
8. Alfirevic Z, Stampalija T, Roberts D, et al. Cervical stitch (cerclage) for preventing preterm birth in singleton pregnancy. Cochrane Database Syst Rev. 2012; 4:CD008991.
9. Ehsanipoor RM, Seligman NS, Saccone G, et al. Physical examination-indicated cerclage: a systematic review and meta-analysis. Obstet Gynecol. 2015;126(1):125-35.
10. Drakeley AJ, Roberts D, Alfirevic Z. Cervical stitch (cerclage) for preventing pregnancy loss in women. Cochrane Database Syst Rev. 2003;1:CD003253.

Chapter 10

Hysteroscopy in Recurrent Pregnancy Loss

Sushma S Deshmukh, Sejal R Naik

Recurrent pregnancy loss
For patient and doctor, it's distress
Difficult to express
Use of hysteroscopy, always yes
As every invention is a worldly creation
Hysteroscopy bloomed up in a stepwise fashion
Accepting critics and honors
Resulting in an extraordinary outcome!

■ INTRODUCTION

Recurrent pregnancy loss (RPL) is one of the most frustrating problems for couples desiring parenthood, and it is often a controversial and confusing clinical challenge for their treating physician. A complete evaluation of couple is not only difficult but yield in the identification of a probable cause in only 40-60% of patients.[1,2]

■ ANATOMICAL CAUSES OF RECURRENT PREGNANCY LOSSES

Approximately 19% of women with at least two or more consecutive miscarriages have uterine anomalies as a causative factor.[2] These can be congenital malformations (bicornuate, didelphic, septate and unicornuate uterus) or acquired defects (fibroids, adenomyosis, adhesions and polyps). In one study, the prevalence of uterine anomalies in patients with RPL is as high as 54.5% and septate uterus is the most common anomaly.[3]

Transvaginal sonography (TVS) is universally considered the initial, noninvasive procedure for assessment of intrauterine pathologies. Hysteroscopy allows for direct visualization, and sampling of the uterine cavity. Since its introduction, hysteroscopy has undergone considerable modifications, leading to an increase in patient compliance and tolerance. Fiberoptics, smaller caliber of the endoscopes, use of simpler distention media, and availability of safer local infiltrative anesthetics have all contributed to the increased use of this technique to evaluate the uterine cavity in the office setting.[4,5]

CONGENITAL UTERINE ANOMALIES

Septate Uterus

Among women with RPL, septate uteri are the most prevalent of the congenital anomalies **(Table 1)**, with prevalence ranges between 1 to 2 per 1,000 and 15 per 1,000 women and its association with RPL is as high as 76%.
A septum may present with the following:
- Infertility
- Spontaneous abortion—50-80% risk
- Preterm labor
- Malpresentation
- Intrauterine growth restriction
- Renal system abnormalities and skeletal abnormalities.

The described pathophysiological mechanism for pregnancy loss in septum is that it prevents proper embryo implantation and development due to poor vascularization. Hysteroscopic resection of a septum is a short outpatient-based surgical procedure with low associated morbidity and has been shown to significantly improve reproductive outcomes. Only 20-25% women with septate uteri have spontaneous abortions and are usually late first or early second trimester miscarriages associated with mini-labors and bleeding. Patients undergoing successful hysteroscopic septum resection seem to enjoy near normal pregnancy outcomes, with term delivery rates of approximately 75% and live birth rates approximating 85%.

Table 1: Prevalence of uterine anomalies among 875 patients with recurrent pregnancy loss.[2]

Uterine anomalies	% occurrence (n)
Total frequency of patients with anomalies	[†]19.3 (169)
Congenital anomalies	7.0 (61)
Bicornuate uterus	0.8 (7)
Didelphic uterus	0.2 (2)
Septate uterus	4.9 (43)
Unicornuate uterus	0.7 (6)
Acquired anomalies[‡]	12.9 (113)
Adhesions	4.1 (36)
Fibroid(s)	6.1 (53)
Polyp(s)	3.1 (27)

[†]Five patients (0.6%) had both congenital and acquired anomalies. These were septum and adhesions, septum and fibroid(s), septum and polyp(s), bicornuate uterus and fibroid(s), and unicornuate uterus and polyp(s). Three patients had a T-shaped uterus.
[‡]Three patients (0.3%) had two acquired anomalies. These were fibroid(s) and polyp(s), adhesions and polyp(s), and adhesions and fibroid(s).[2]

Classification

Uterine septum is classified into two types as complete septate uterus and partial or subseptate uterus. A septum can be called as complete septum if it extends from the fundus of the uterus to the internal os.

- American Society for Reproductive Medicine (ASRM) in 1988 classified septate uterus as class V (Va complete and Vb partial) and suggested an internal fundal indentation length equal or greater than 1 cm.[6]
- European Society of Human Reproduction and Embryology–European Society for Gynaecological Endoscopy (ESHRE-ESGE) in 2013 classified septate uterus as class U2. Septate uterus is defined as an internal indentation at the fundus in the midline with greater than 50% myometrial thickness. Class U2 is further divided into Class U2a or partial septate uterus and class U2b complete septate uterus.[7]

It is important to note that the septate uterus can be associated with a double cervix and a double cervix with vaginal septum.

ASRM (2016) radiologically defines:
- *Normal/arcuate*: Depth from the interstitial line to the apex of the indentation is <1 cm and angle of indentation >90°.
- *Septate:* Depth from the interstitial line to the apex of the indentation >1.5 cm and angle of the indentation <90° **(Figs. 1A and B)**.

Diagnosis

Investigative modalities available for diagnosis are as follows:
- *Ultrasound [Transvaginal ultrasonography, hysterosonography, and three-dimensional ultrasonography (3D-US)]:* Ultrasound is an indispensable and sensitive tool with sensitivity of ranges between 95.21% and 99.29%.[8]

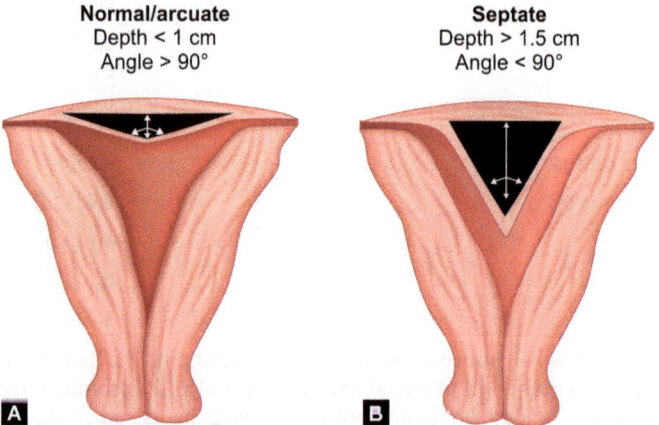

Figs. 1A and B: (A) Normal/arcuate; and (B) Septate uterus.

The estimated accuracy of 3D-US in the diagnosis of uterine malformation is as high as 91.6% in the study of the external uterine contour and 100% in that of the cavity **(Fig. 2)**.[9]

- *Hysterosalpingography (HSG)*: HSG provides the graphical record of the uterine cavity. In cases of uterine septum, the imaging shows smaller than normal symmetric endometrial cavities. There can be confusion in diagnosing a septate and bicornuate uterus. If the angle of divergence of two straight uterine cavities is 75° or less, it indicates the presence of a septate uterus **(Fig. 3)**. Limitations of HSG include the lack of information about the contour of the uterus, exposure to ionizing radiation, and the risk of reproductive tract infection.
- *Magnetic resonance imaging*: There is an excellent correlation between MRI and clinical diagnosis of müllerian anomalies. Its major advantage is the high soft tissue resolution. But it is not cost-effective.

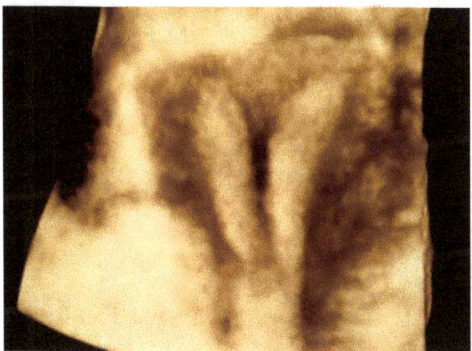

Fig. 2: Ultrasonography picture of septate uterus.
Courtesy: Dr Ravi Kadasane.

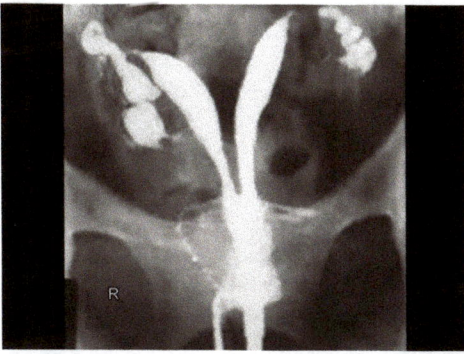

Fig. 3: Hysterosalpingography showing septate uterus.
Courtesy: Dr Sandeep Mahajan.

- *Laparoscopy/Hysteroscopy* **(Figs. 4 and 5)**: The combination of hysteroscopy and laparoscopy is complementary to each other and considered as the "gold standard" for the diagnosis of uterine malformation. But they cannot be used as a primary tool. The advantage is the confirmation of diagnosis and correction in the same sitting, i.e. "See and Treat".

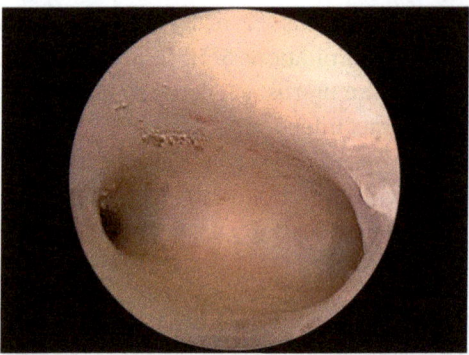

Fig. 4: Normal uterine cavity.

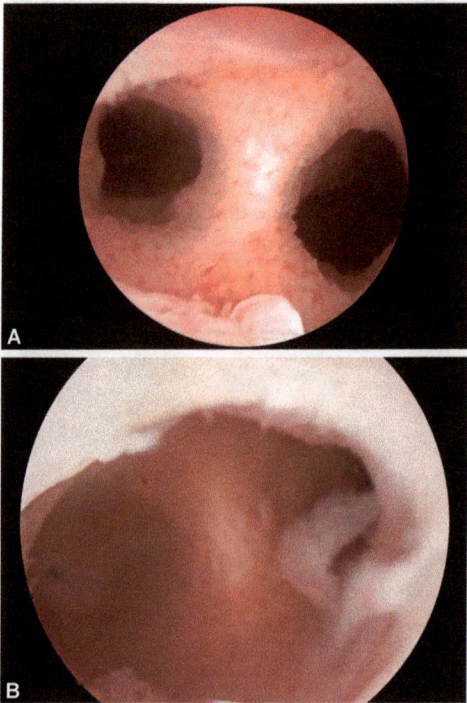

Figs. 5A and B: (A) Complete septate uterus; (B) Subseptate uterus.

Methods of Surgical Treatment

The gold standard method for treatment is hysteroscopic metroplasty which can be done by division or incision of the uterine septum using cold scissors, electrosurgery, resectoscope with an operating loop, laser. The best time to perform metroplasty is the early proliferative phase. Misoprostol is an effective ripening agent to induce adequate cervical dilatation prior to septum resection.[10]

Office hysteroscopy: It can be done in an office environment with a diameter 2.9 mm or smaller telescope, 4.5 mm inner sheath and 5 mm outer sheath, and 5 fr scissors can be introduced from working channel **(Fig. 6)**. It can be introduced into the uterine cavity without dilatation of cervix with continuous flow vaginoscopy. Moving the hysteroscope from side to side and visualization of both the ostia on a panoramic view from the level of internal os verifies the completion of resection.

Practical points:
- Normal saline is commonly used as distension media for diagnostic hysteroscopy as well as with bipolar energy in operative procedures. Glycine is used when monopolar energy is employed. Ideal light source is xenon and camera is high definition.
- Width of the septum is judged by opening the jaws of the scissors which is 6 mm **(Fig. 7)**. If the width is more than 10 mm, it is better to use electrodes.

Resectoscope: It needs a 4 mm telescope with operative sheath with a diameter of 7–8.5 mm. The cervix will need a dilatation of 10 mm. The procedure is performed with monopolar or bipolar energy and using a Collins loop/knife. Recently, mini-resectoscopes with small diameters have been developed avoiding the needed for cervical dilatation. Metroplasty can be performed in an office setting. It is advisable to perform a diagnostic hysteroscopy first. Once the diagnosis is confirmed, resection is performed using right-angled knife.

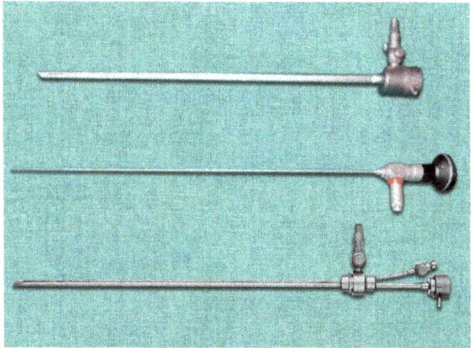

Fig. 6: Bettocchi's 2.9 mm hysteroscope and 5 mm operative sheath.

Usually a monopolar underwater cutting current of 80–120 W is sufficient for performing the septum resection. Strict account of intake and output of glycine should be maintained.

Bipolar and monopolar resectoscopic loops were compared in one randomized study and showed similar efficacy and safety. Once the satisfactory resection of the septum **(Figs. 8A and B)** is performed, the hysteroscopic

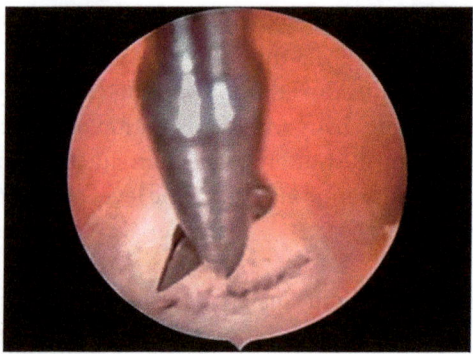

Fig. 7: Resection of septum.

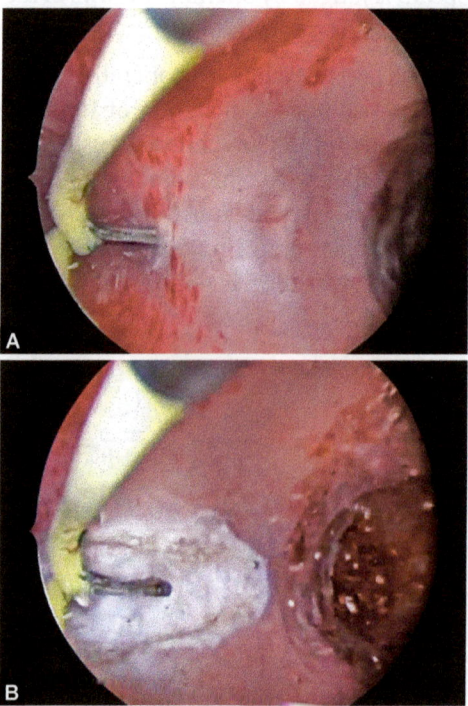

Figs. 8A and B: Resection of septum with resectoscope.

assembly is withdrawn and hemostasis is confirmed. Bleeding following the procedure is self-limiting or may require uterine bimanual massage.

Postoperative Care

- Antibiotics
- *Prevention of intrauterine adhesions*: Adhesion prevention is not needed in subseptal resection procedures. In complete septum, adhesion prevention can be done with Foley's catheter of size 8 (balloon distended with 3 cc saline), intrauterine instillation of hyaluronic acid or inserting an intrauterine device.
- Two cycles of estradiol valerate 2 mg TDS for 21 days along with oral progesterone 10 mg once a day from day 16 to 25 are used for rapid epithelization and endometrial proliferation over the resected raw area to prevent adhesions.
- About 7–10% of patients develop intrauterine adhesions especially at the fundus which may mimic the residual septum. Imaging modality is used for confirming the result after 2 months. It is well accepted after the study of Fedele that women with a residual septum <1 cm shown by ultrasonography after the hysteroscopic metroplasty does not affect the reproductive outcome compared to women with a complete resection.[11]
- In selected group of patients, second look hysteroscopy is advocated 8 weeks following the resection of the septum.

Complications

Complication following septum resection is uncommon:
- Perforation of the uterus
- Postoperative bleeding
- Rarely fluid overload.

Bicornuate Uteri

Bicornuate uteri are associated with a similar increase in miscarriage rate among women with RPL (86%), although bicornuate anomalies are much less common. There is no strong evidence that surgical repair reduces the miscarriage rate for women with RPL who have bicornuate uterine defects.[12]

Unicornuate Uterus

This anomaly results from complete or near-complete arrested development of one of the müllerian ducts **(Figs. 9A to C)**. Four possible subtypes can develop: (1) absent rudimentary horn, (2) noncavitary (nonfunctional) rudimentary horn, (3) cavitary communicating rudimentary horn, and

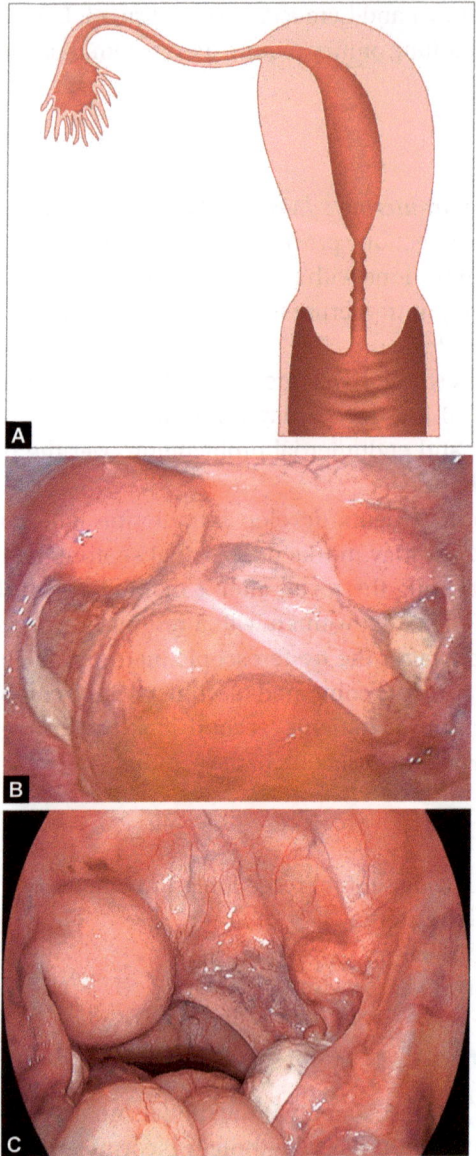

Figs. 9A to C: Unicornuate uterus.

(4) cavitary noncommunicating rudimentary horn. The last one may obstruct and present with abdominal pain, subsequently requiring surgical intervention.

Although a patient with a unicornuate uterus can have a normal pregnancy, spontaneous abortion rates range between 41% and 62% and premature birth rates range between 10% and 20%. Other complications include abnormal fetal lie and intrauterine growth restriction.[3] Lateral

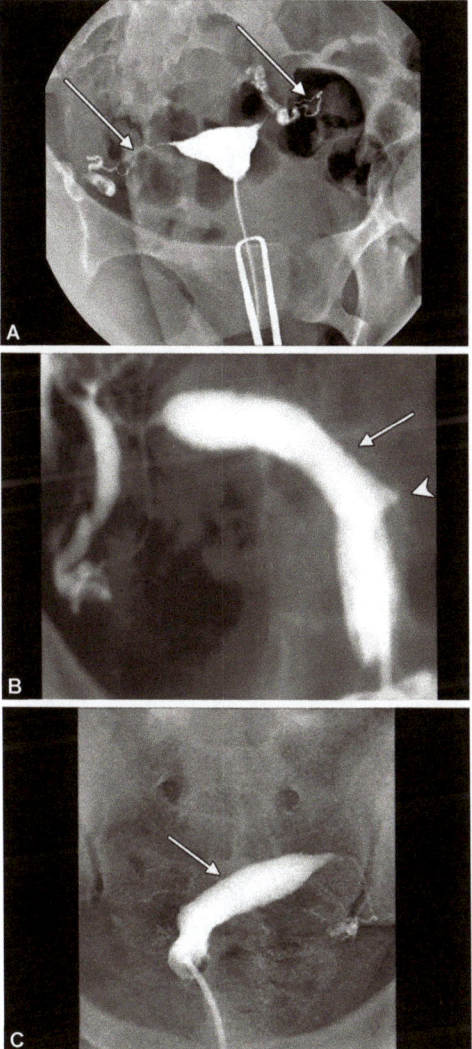

Figs. 10A to C: Normal uterine cavity in hysterosalpingography (HSG), unicornuate uterus with normal ipsilateral tube in HSG.

metroplasty by hysteroscopy to improve neonatal outcome can be tried with guarded response in recurrent preterm births **(Figs. 10 to 12)**.

Pregnancy implanting in the rudimentary horn usually has a disastrous outcome, with most resulting in uterine rupture.[1,3]

■ ACQUIRED UTERINE ANOMALIES

In contrast to congenital uterine defects, acquired uterine anomalies develop in response to hormonal or physical stimuli experienced after puberty; and in

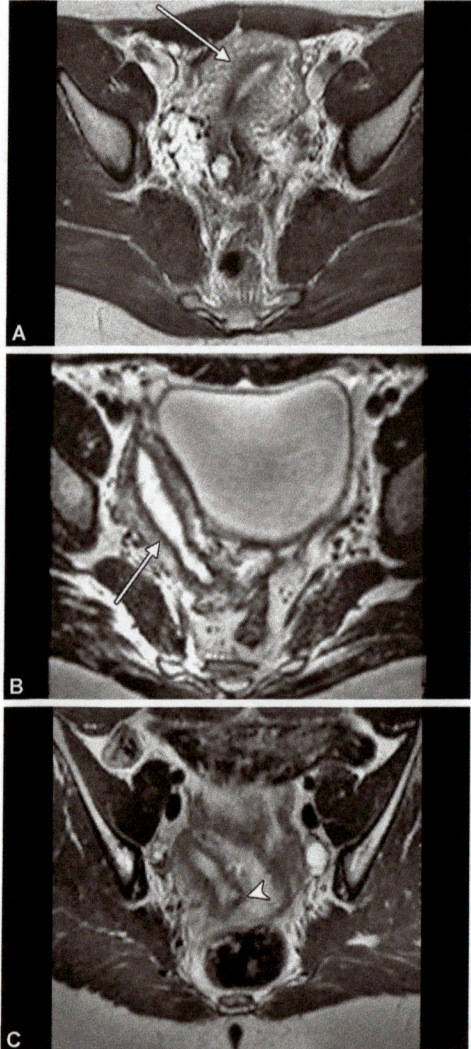

Figs. 11A to C: Class II unicornuate uterus with no rudimentary horn. Arrows show classic banana shape appearance of the unicornuate uterus.

women with RPL, they are almost twice as prevalent as congenital anomalies (*see* **Table 1**).

Intrauterine Adhesions

The intrauterine adhesions typically form after endometrial trauma, often as a result of curettage following abortions, which may exacerbate the problem in women with RPL. It may involve different layers of the endometrium, myometrium, or connective tissue, thus leading to implantation failure and

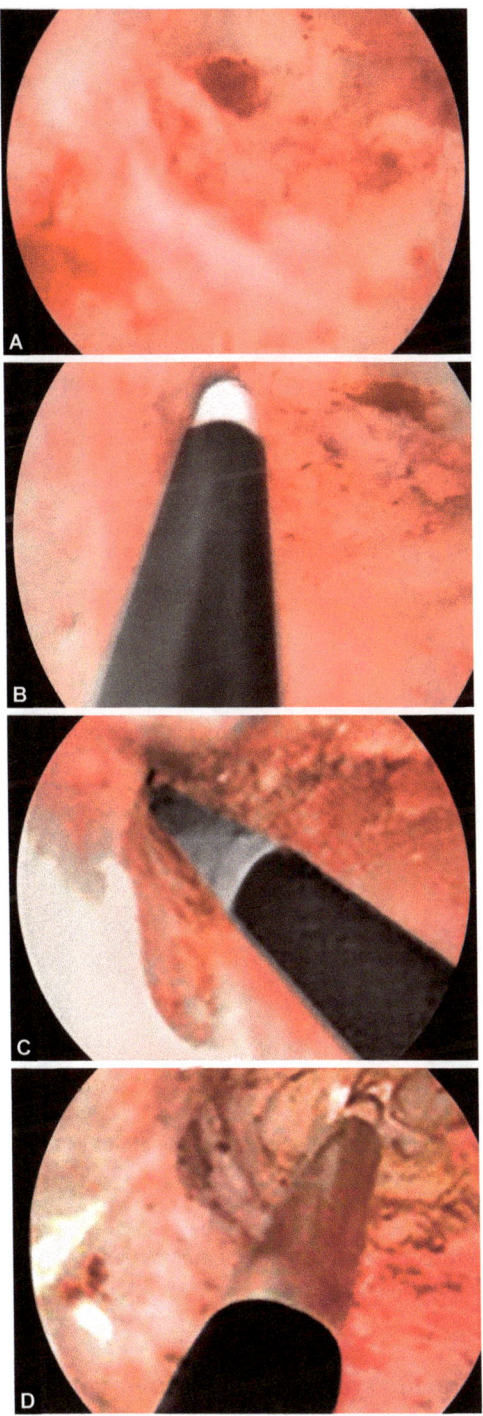

Figs. 12A to D

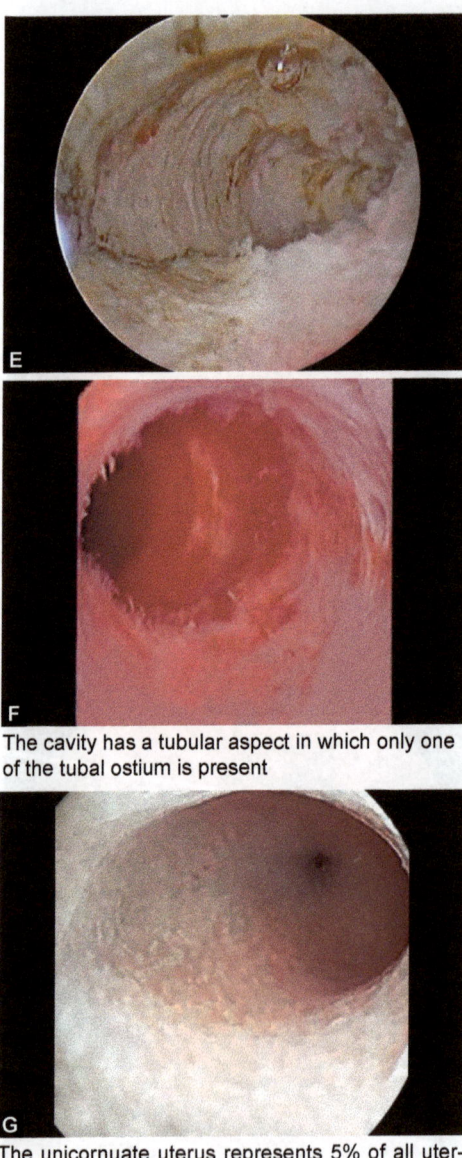

The cavity has a tubular aspect in which only one of the tubal ostium is present

The unicornuate uterus represents 5% of all uterine malformations that translates in one in 4020 women

Figs. 12E to G

Figs. 12A to G: Hysteroscopic view of unicornuate uterus and lateral metroplasty. *Courtesy:* Dr Sunita Tandulwadkar.

miscarriages. Asherman's syndrome (AS) causes endometrial fibrosis. The distinction between the functional and basal layers of the endometrium is lost, and the fibrotic adhesion forms across the cavity.

Hysteroscopy is now the gold standard of diagnosis and treatment since it provides a good view of the cavity, allowing a precise description of the location and degree of adhesions and concurrent treatment of adhesions. In one review, women with adhesions experienced a high rate of miscarriages (40%) compared with women who had surgical adhesiolysis (25%).[13] However, the extent of endometrial fibrosis will determine the reproductive outcome after an anatomic restoration of the uterus. A thin endometrium that fails to respond to hormones leads to implantation failure or early miscarriages due to lack of blood supply **(Figs. 13 to 15)**.

Standard Procedure

Either monopolar needle/scissors/versa point/Collin's knife is used to release adhesions. One should withdraw the scope till internal os from time to time, to have a panoramic view of cavity for orientation and to avoid going in the

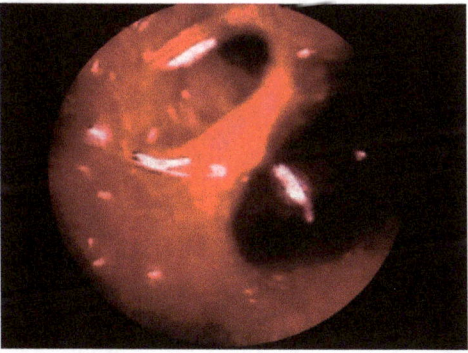

Fig. 13: Fine and fragile endometrial synechiae.
Courtesy: Dr Sunita Tandulwadkar.

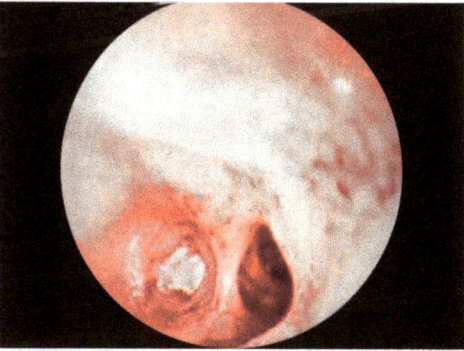

Fig. 14: Myofibrous synechiae near to tubal ostium, remaining endometrium is atrophic.
Courtesy: Dr Sunita Tandulwadkar.

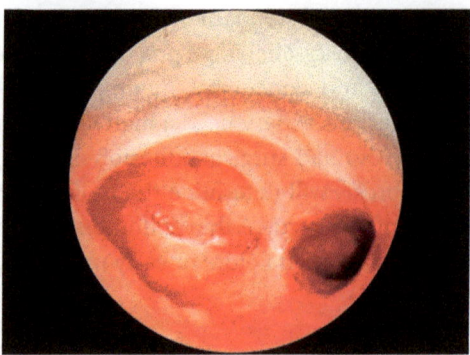

Fig. 15: Connective tissue synechiae with partial debridement.
Courtesy: Dr Sunita Tandulwadkar.

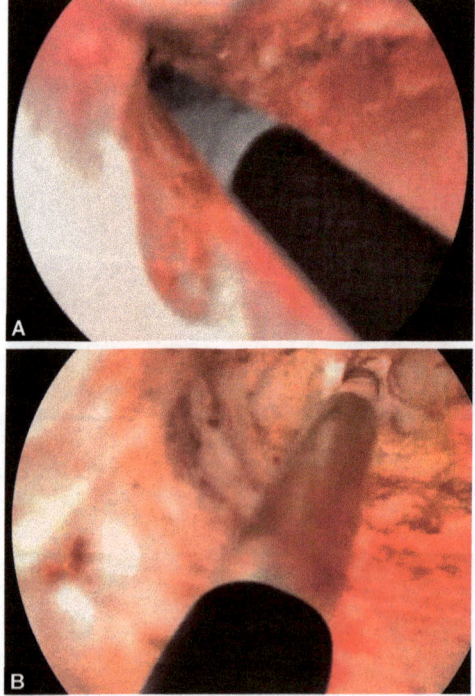

Figs. 16A and B: With versa scope lateral and vertical strokes taken so as to release adhesions.
Courtesy: Dr Sunita Tandulwadkar.

wrong plane. Adhesiolysis should be stopped once the pink myometrium is reached. Good intrauterine pressure should be maintained. Postoperative estrogen and progesterone treatment for 4–6 weeks is advisable to enhance endometrial growth **(Figs. 16 to 19)**.

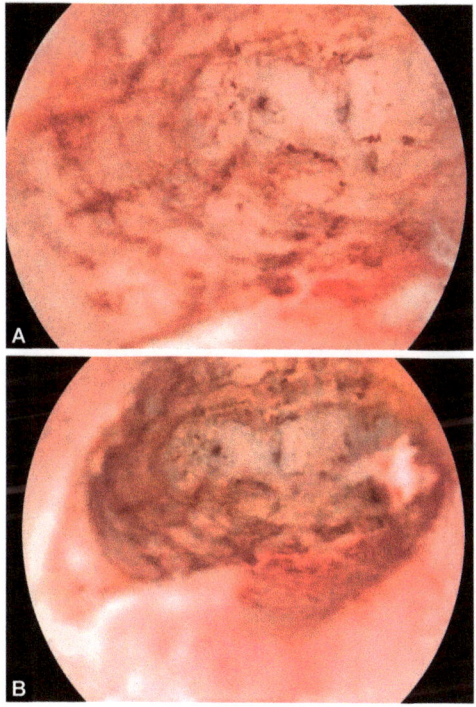

Figs. 17A and B: End result (nearly normal cavity).
Courtesy: Dr Sunita Tandulwadkar.

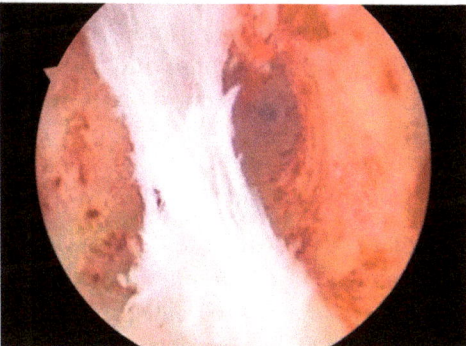

Fig. 18: Band of intrauterine adhesions at isthmus can easily be released with scissors.
Courtesy: Dr Sunita Tandulwadkar.

Fibroids

The prevalence of submucosal and cavity-distorting myomas in women with two or more pregnancy losses was found to be 4.08%.[14] The prevalence of uterine myomas was highest in women with three or more RPLs (5.91%).[14]

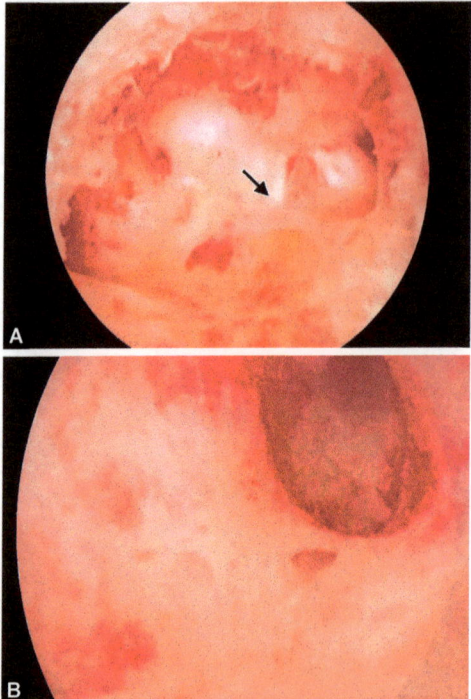

Figs. 19A and B: Filmy adhesions in cavity and near cornu.
Courtesy: Dr Sunita Tandulwadkar.

Submucosal fibroids, type 0 and I fibroids are those most amenable to hysteroscopic resection. It should be performed during the follicular phase to ensure that the patient is not pregnant and for optimal visualization. Generally, fibroids are more likely to contribute to RPL if they distort the endometrial cavity and/or are >6 cm.

Standard Procedure (Figs. 20 to 22)

Either unipolar or bipolar resectoscope can be used with following settings: Flow rate of approximately 250 mL/minute, pressure of 80–100 mm Hg, monopolar electricity generator at 60–100 watts, and suction pressure of 0.25 bars. Fluid balance is recorded by measuring the infused and drained fluid from continuous flow resectoscope.

Myoma is shaved down with slicing technique. Type I and type II myomas are shaved down to the level of myometrium till myoma becomes flat. After that the removal of the part nested deep in the myometrial wall can be achieved by two techniques:

1. Hydromassage can be done by opening and closing the endouterine aspiration system. Myoma will start protruding into the cavity which can be sliced off. The myoma may be removed in a single sitting.

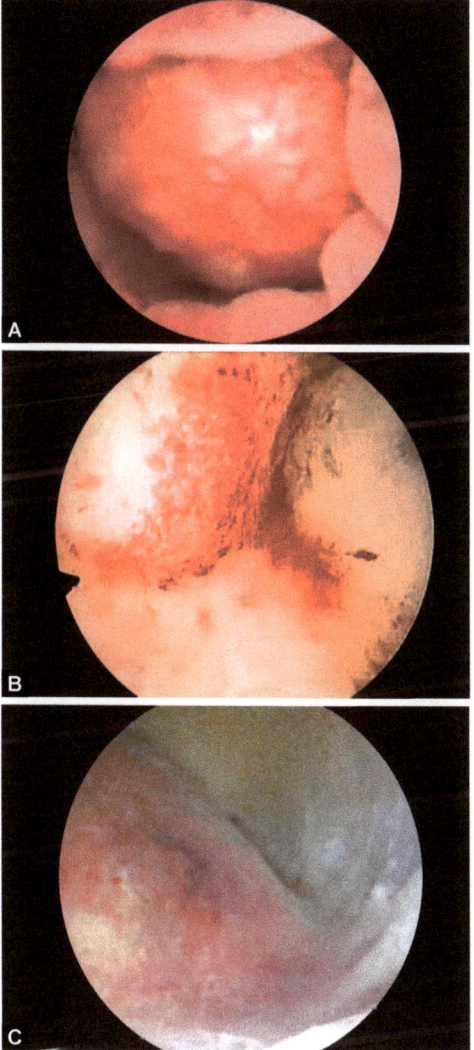

Figs. 20A to C: Type 0, 1, and 2 myomas.
Courtesy: Dr Sunita Tandulwadkar (Figs. A and B) and Dr Paul PG (Fig. C).

2. *Cold-knife technique*: It consists of simple, mechanical passage of the resectoscope loop along the capsule lining of the myoma, detaching it from the fibrous bridges that anchor it to the uterine wall without any electrocoagulation.

If it is impossible to totally remove the intramural fibroid in one sitting, the fibroid can be removed at a later date (after 2–3 months). Intramural component of the myoma is known to migrate into the uterine cavity.

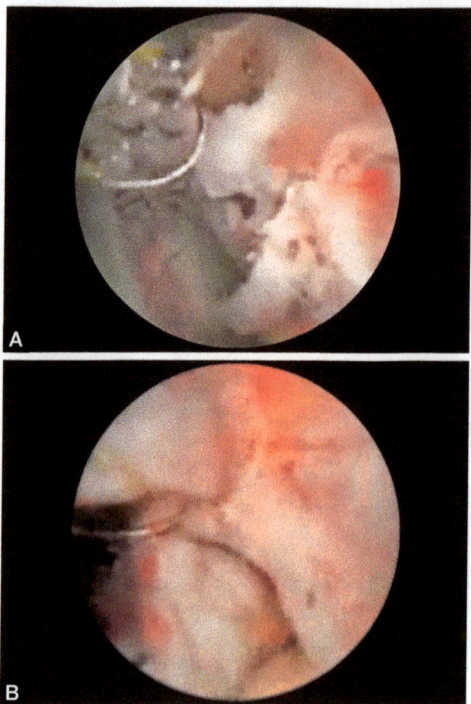

Figs. 21A and B: Resection of type 0 myoma.
Courtesy: Dr Sunita Tandulwadkar.

Meticulous attention to intraoperative fluid balance is imperative. If fluid deficit of more than 1–1.5 L is detected, serum sodium level is measured and hyponatremia, if present, should be treated. For every liter of electrolyte free fluid that is absorbed the sodium will go down approximately 10 mEq/L. This helps surgeon to determine when to stop a case. If deficit is approximately 1,500 cc, it is advisable to put in a Foley's catheter and give diuretic. Myomectomy of large myomas is liable to hyponatremia, hypo-osmolality, increased central venous pressure, increased prothrombin time and activated partial thromboplastin time, and increase of most of the cardiodynamic parameters. It is advisable not to remove big anterior and posterior fibroids in the same sitting to avoid intrauterine adhesions/synechiae formations.

Polyps

Polyps are hormonally-induced growths of the endometrium. Research is lacking regarding the role of polyps in pregnancy loss. For polyps, surgical removal is often considered for women with RPL if no other causes for pregnancy loss have been found **(Figs. 23 and 24)**.

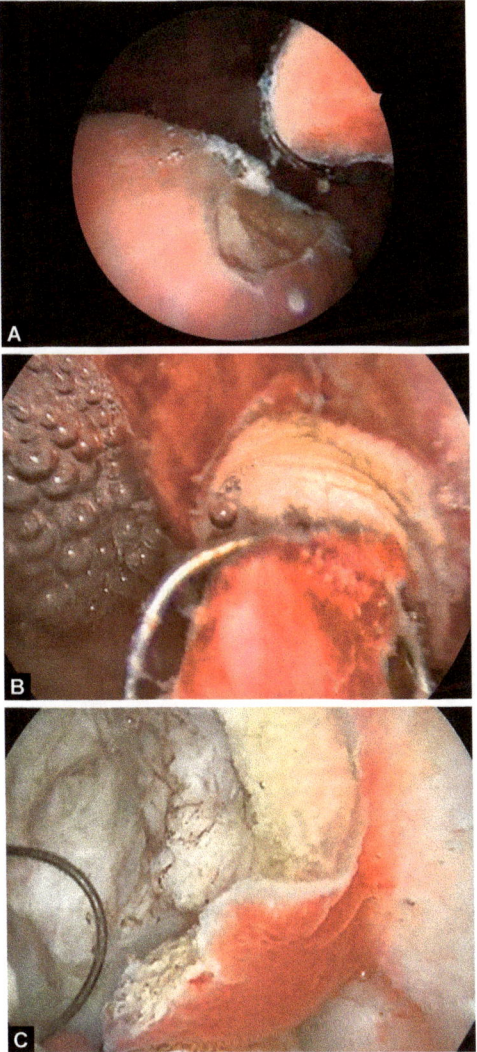

Figs. 22A to C: Resection of myoma with loop electrode.
Courtesy: Dr Paul PG.

Adenomas

They are overgrowths of the glandular endometrium within the muscular myometrium; if large, they can cause the same distortion of the endometrial cavity seen with fibroids and thus possibly contribute to RPL. The presence of adenomyosis can increase the risk of miscarriage and reduce the likelihood of delivering a viable baby by overall 30%.[15] This rise in miscarriage rate is

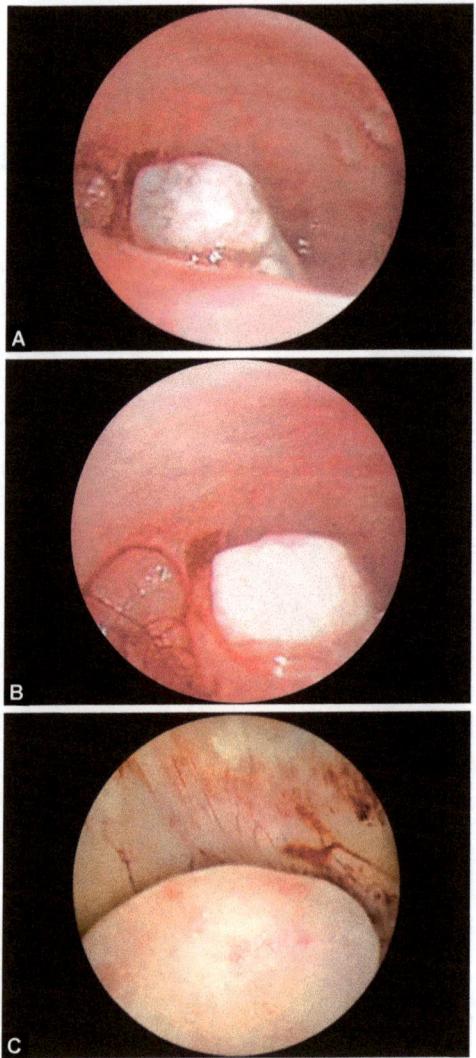

Figs. 23A to C: Endometrial polyp.
Courtesy: Dr Sunita Tandulwadkar (Figs. A and B) and Dr Paul PG (Fig. C).

observed in donor cycles too, i.e. it is independent of oocyte and embryo quality.[16]

Hysteroscopy is more specific but less sensitive in diagnosis of adenomyosis. One can see variety of presentation with adenomyosis and hence subjected to under/over reporting. There may be irregular endometrium, endometrial defects. About 50% of cases have an abnormal hypervascularization and cystic hemorrhagic lesions with brownish fluid **(Figs. 25 and 26)**.

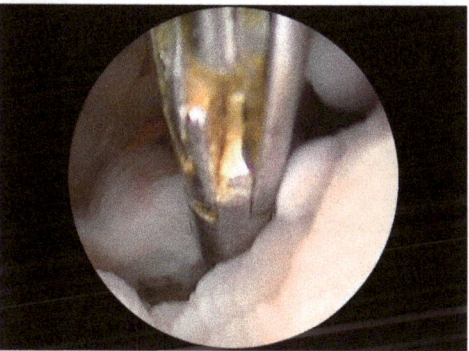

Fig. 24: Hysteroscopic polypectomy using polypectomy forceps.
Courtesy: Dr Paul PG.

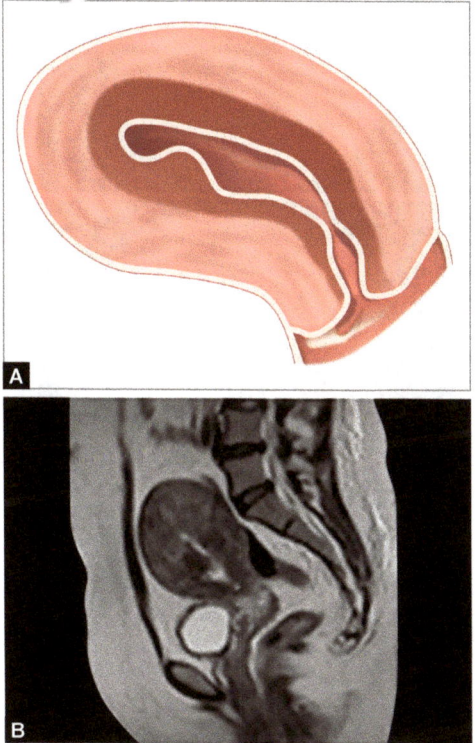

Figs. 25A and B

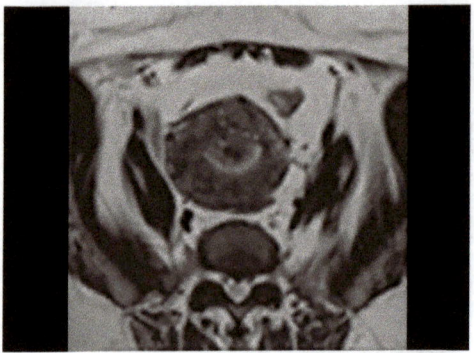

Fig. 25C

Figs. 25A to C: Pictorial presentation and MRI findings of polypoidal adenomyoma.
Courtesy: Dr Sunita Tandulwadkar.

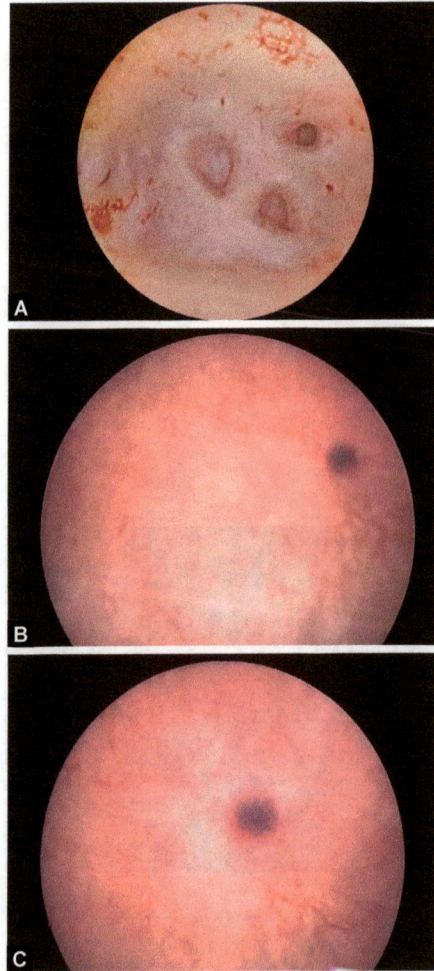

Figs. 26A to C

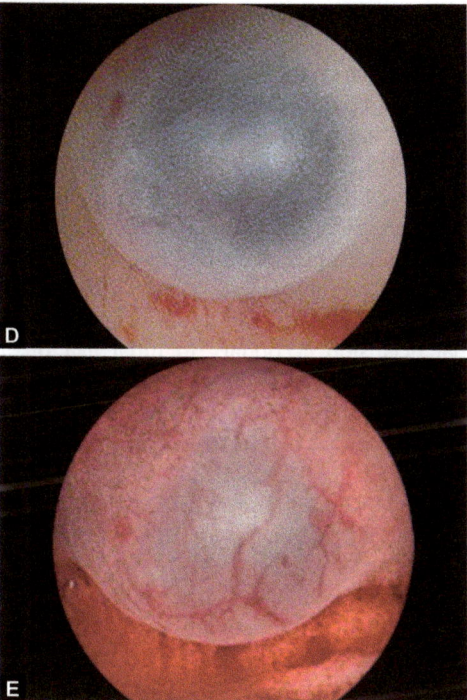

Figs. 26D and E

Figs. 26A to E: Hysteroscopic findings of adenomyosis, punctations, hemorrhagic cysts, and blebs.
Courtesy: Dr Sunita Tandulwadkar.

■ CONCLUSION

Anatomic abnormalities, both acquired and congenital, account for about 20% of the explainable causes of RPL. Minimally invasive surgery is suitable for correction of most of these abnormalities. In general, pregnancy rates are significantly improved after surgical correction.

■ ACKNOWLEDGMENTS

Dr Sushma S Deshmukh, Dr Sejal R Naik, Dr Paul PG, Dr Sunita Tandulwadkar, Dr Ravi Kadasane, and Dr Sandeep Mahajan.

■ REFERENCES

1. Brezina PR, Kutteh WH. Classic and cutting-edge strategies for the management of early pregnancy loss. Obstet Gynecol Clin North Am. 2014;41:1-18.
2. Jaslow CR, Carney JL, Kutteh WH. Diagnostic factors identified in 1020 women with two verses three or more recurrent pregnancy losses. Fertil Steril. 2010;93:1234-44.

3. Elsokkary M, Elshourbagy M, Labib K, et al. Assessment of hysteroscopic role in management of women with recurrent pregnancy loss. J Matern Fetal Neonatal Med. 2018;31(11):1494-504.
4. Pal L, Lapensee L, Toth TL, et al. Comparison of office hysteroscopy, transvaginal ultrasonography and endometrial biopsy in evaluation of abnormal uterine bleeding. JSLS. 1997;1(2):125-30.
5. Katke RD, Zarariya AN. Use of diagnostic hysteroscopy in abnormal uterine bleeding in perimenopausal age group and its clinicopathological co-relation with ultrasound and histopathology findings: experience in a tertiary care institute. Int J Reprod Contracept Obstet Gynecol. 2015;4(2):413-8.
6. The American Fertility Society classifications of adnexal adhesions, distal tubal occlusion, tubal occlusion secondary to tubal ligation, tubal pregnancies, müllerian anomalies and intrauterine adhesions. Fertil Steril. 1988;49:944-55.
7. Grimbizis GF, Gordts S, Di SpiezioSardo A, et al. The ESHRE-ESGE consensus on the classification of female genital tract congenital anomalies. Gynecol Surg. 2013;10(3):199-212.
8. Mueller GC, Hussain HK, Smith YR, et al. Müllerian duct anomalies: comparison of MRI diagnosis and clinical diagnosis. American Journal of Roentgenology. 2007;189(6):1294-302.
9. Raga F, Bonilla-Musoles F, Blanes J, et al. Congenital müllerian anomalies: diagnostic accuracy of three-dimensional ultrasound. Fertil Steril. 1996;65(3):523-8.
10. Kamel Mostafa AM, El-Tawab Sally S, El-Ashkar Osama S, et al. Mini-scissor versus bipolar twizzle in ambulatory hysteroscopic metroplasty: a prospective randomized study. J Gynecol Surg. 2014;30(3):147-51.
11. Fedele L, Bianchi S, Marchini M, et al. Residual uterine septum of less than 1 cm after hysteroscopic metroplasty does not impair reproductive outcome. Hum Reprod. 1996;11(4):727-9.
12. Sugiura-Ogasawara M, Lin BL, Aoki K, et al. Does surgery improve live birth rates in patients with recurrent miscarriage caused by uterine anomalies? J Obstet Gynaecol. 2014;24:1-4.
13. Schenker JG, Margalioth EJ. Intrauterine adhesions: an updated appraisal. Fertil Steril. 1982;37:593-610.
14. Russo M, Suen M, Bedaiwy M, et al. Prevalence of uterine myomas among women with 2 or more recurrent pregnancy losses: a systematic review. J Minim Invasive Gynecol. 2016;23(5):702-6.
15. Vercellini P, Consonni D, Dridi D, et al. Uterine adenomyosis and in vitro fertilization outcome: a systematic review and meta-analysis. Hum Reprod. 2014;29(5):964-77.
16. Park CW, Choi MH, Yang KM, et al. Pregnancy rate in women with adenomyosis undergoing fresh or frozen embryo transfer cycles following gonadotropin-releasing hormone agonist treatment. Clin Exp Reprod Med. 2016;43(3):169-73.

Chapter 11

Role of Male Factor in Recurrent Pregnancy Loss

Ruchi Pathak

■ INTRODUCTION

We are still unsure about the exact etiology of recurrent pregnancy loss (RPL) with 50% cases being labeled as those with an unknown etiology.[1] Even among the known causes and despite the fact that sperm integrity is essential for sperm-egg interactions, fertilization and early embryonic development[2-4] and the proliferation and invasiveness of trophoblast cells being under the regulation of paternally expressed genes,[5-7] the current focus in a couple with RPL is mainly on the female factors.[1]

The focus has shifted to male factors contributing to RPL only recently. Male factors that may contribute to RPL are discussed in the chapter.

■ CHROMOSOMAL ABNORMALITIES

Recent studies point toward chromosomal abnormalities of spermatozoa as one of the causative factors for RPL.

Fluorescence in situ hybridization (FISH) analysis allows sperm exhibiting abnormalities in motility or other aspects of fertilization to be assessed by chromosome-specific DNA probes. Though the number of chromosomes probed at any one time is limited, hundreds of sperms may be analyzed by this technique.

- *Sperm aneuploidy*: An increased incidence of sperm aneuploidy is observed in men with oligospermia, as the sperm concentration drops below 10 million/mL.[8-10] Meiotic studies in men with nonobstructive azoospermia, using immunocytogenetic techniques, have demonstrated errors of chromosome synapsis and significantly reduced recombination. An increased risk of aneuploidy in sperm surgically removed from testes is observed in these men.
- *Chromosome microdeletions and duplications*: There seems to be a possibility of lethal chromosomal duplications or microdeletions contributing to pregnancy loss. The possibility is raised by the presence of a significant minority of euploid embryos at the time of hysteroscopic observation before performing suction and evacuation in cases of missed abortions. Simultaneous evaluation of all chromosomes can be

done by comparative genome hybridization (CGH). It can also identify submicroscopic copy number variations in a whole genome imbalance in immature germ cells. In a study by Ivanka et al. in six men, all analyzed men had copy number variations in sperm DNA (using microarray-based CGH, ejaculates of six males with idiopathic azoospermia and normal karyotype). In 5 out of 6 patients (83.3%), the most consistent were aberrations in Y-chromosome. The mechanism of embryonic loss due to the genetic alteration is yet to be explored.

- *RPL due to environmental toxins*: The process of normal spermatogenesis is disrupted by a wide variety of toxicants present in environment such as pesticides, metals, and air pollutants. A significant increase in chromosome breaks was observed in individuals with occupational exposure to benzene in the study carried out by Marchetti et al. in Tianjin, China.

■ EPIGENETICS

Epigenetics is the study of heritable phenotypic changes in organisms that is not due to alteration in underlying DNA sequence. Epigenetic structure of sperm DNA seems to play an important role in normal function of sperm gamete and embryo development. During normal spermiogenesis, nuclear histone is replaced by Protamine 1 and 2 in ratio of approximately 1:1. An abnormal P1/P2 ratio has been associated with reduced sperm concentration, abnormal sperm morphology, increased sperm DNA fragmentation, and reduced fertilization and implantation rates.[11] The regulation of DNA methylation is essential to the normal function of gamete and embryo development.[11] Gene activation occurs due to increased accessibility of DNA by polymerase. This gene activation occurs by hypomethylation. On the other hand, gene expression is inhibited by hypermethylation as it blocks access of DNA by polymerase. Some methylation defects in sperm can be corrected by oocyte depending depends on the quality of the egg, and level of abnormality of methylation.

■ RECURRENT PREGNANCY LOSS DUE TO OXIDATIVE STRESS AND DNA DAMAGE

Human spermatozoa are vulnerable to free radical attack by reactive oxygen species such as superoxide anions, hydrogen peroxide leading to oxidative DNA damage resulting in DNA strand breaks.[11] DNA damage has been linked to chemotherapy and radiotherapy, cigarette smoking, varicocele, hyperthermia, and aging.[12] High content of polyunsaturated fatty acid in sperm plasma membrane, limited cytoplasmic volume makes it vulnerable to oxidative stress. Sperm is, therefore, dependent on antioxidants present in male reproductive tract secretions. In cases of males who smoke, DNA in sperm nucleus is damaged but the sperm is able to fertilize the oocyte. While egg cytoplasm has the ability to repair damaged DNA, this ability may vary between individual eggs and between women of different age.[11]

There is an association between sperm DNA fragmentation and RPL. However, given the significant heterogeneity between various studies and lack of prospective pregnancy outcome data, further large prospective studies are needed to establish the association.[13]

■ ANTISPERM ANTIBODIES

Exposure of the antigens present on the surface of the developing sperms in the male testes with blood components may occur because of infection, chemical or physical injury. This may trigger the development of antisperm antibodies which may adversely affect the motility, morphology, and the penetrating capacity of the sperm. It has been postulated that the presence of antisperm antibodies may be associated with immune rejection of the embryo.

■ ROLE OF SEMINAL FLUID IN RECURRENT PREGNANCY LOSS

Seminal fluid is not only a transport medium for the sperm but also facilitates the implantation of embryo within the endometrium. It contains a number of chemicals which include high content of TGF-beta[14] and PGE prostaglandins,[15] and many other factors like cytokines,[16] prostasomes,[17] and polyamines,[18] etc. which work as modulators of female immune system so that the embryo can be protected from damage by the maternal immune system and develop normally through a state of active immune tolerance. Any imbalance in the constituent of seminal fluid may thus have an adverse impact on the developing embryo.

■ PATERNAL AGE

The absence of a universal definition for advanced paternal age makes its effect on quality of semen and reproductive function difficult to correlate. The studies on paternal age impact on successful pregnancy outcome shows conflicting results.[19]

Advanced paternal age however is associated with increase in incidence of genetic diseases.[19] The exhaustive literature review has demonstrated negative effects on sperm quality and testicular functions with increasing paternal age.[19] Epigenetics changes, DNA mutations along with chromosomal aneuploidies have been associated with increasing paternal age.[19]

CONCLUSION

The various changes in the male reproductive system that may contribute to RPL have been elucidated in this chapter. A clear understanding of the causes and the management options still remain elusive. More research is needed to comprehend the contribution of the male towards RPL. This will lead to treatment options of this perplexing condition.

REFERENCES

1. Practice Committee of the American Society for Reproductive Medicine. Evaluation and treatment of recurrent pregnancy loss: a committee opinion. Fertil Steril. 2012;98:1103-11.
2. Simerly C, Wu GJ, Zoran S, et al. The paternal inheritance of the centrosome, the cell's microtubule-organizing center, in humans, and the implications for infertility. Nat Med. 1995;1:47-52.
3. Van Blerkom J. Sperm centrosome dysfunction: a possible new class of male factor infertility in the human. Mol Hum Reprod. 1996;2:349-54.
4. Moomjy M, Colombero LT, Veeck LL, et al. Sperm integrity is critical for normal mitotic division and early embryonic development. Mol Hum Reprod. 1999;5: 836-44.
5. Janny L, Menezo YJ. Evidence for a strong paternal effect on human preimplantation embryo development and blastocyst formation. Mol Reprod Dev. 1994;38:36-42.
6. Check JH, Katsoff D, Check ML. Some semen abnormalities may cause infertility by impairing implantation rather than fertilization. Med Hypotheses. 2001;56:653-7.
7. Goshen R, Ben-Rafael Z, Gonik B, et al. The role of genomic imprinting in implantation. Fertil Steril. 1994;62:903-10.
8. Sun F, Ko E, Martin RH. Is there a relationship between sperm chromatin abnormalities and sperm morphology? Reprod Biol Endocrinol. 2006;4:1.
9. Templado C, Lroz L, Estop A. New insights on the origin and relevance of aneuploidy in human spermatozoa. Mol Hum Reprod. 2013;16:634-43.
10. Martin RH, Rademaker AW, Greene C, et al. A comparison of the frequency of sperm chromosome abnormalities in men with mild, moderate, and severe oligozoospermia. Biol Reprod. 2003;69:535-9.
11. Jenkins TG, Carrell DT. The sperm epigenome and potential implications for the developing embryo. Reproduction. 2012;143:727-34.
12. Aitken RJ, Baker MA. Causes and consequences of apoptosis in spermatozoa; contributions to infertility and impacts on development. Int J Dev Biol. 2013;57:265-72.
13. McQueen DB, Zhang J, Robins JC. Sperm DNA fragmentation and recurrent pregnancy loss: a systematic review and meta-analysis. Fertil Steril. 2019;112(1):54-60.
14. Robertson SA, Ingman WV, O'Leary S, et al. Transforming growth factor beta—A mediator of immune deviation in seminal plasma. J Reprod Immunol. 2002;57:109-28.

15. Kelly RW. Prostaglandins in primate semen: Biasing the immune system to benefit spermatozoa and virus? Prostaglandins Leukot Essent Fatty Acids. 1997;57:113-8.
16. Maegawa M, Kanada M, Irahara M, et al. A repertoire of cytokines in human seminal plasma. J Reprod Immunol. 2002;54:33-42.
17. Burden HP, Holmes CBH, Persad R, et al. Prostasomes: Their effects on human male reproduction and fertility. Hum Reprod Update. 2006;12:283-92.
18. Shohat B, Maayan R, Singer M, et al. Immunosuppressive activity and polyamine levels of seminal plasma in azoospermic, oligospermic, and normospermic men. Arch Androl. 1990;24:41-50.
19. Sharma R, Agarwal A, Rohra VK, et al. Effects of increased paternal age on sperm quality, reproductive outcome and associated epigenetic risks to offspring. Reprod Biol Endocrinol. 2015;13:35.

Chapter 12

Infections and Recurrent Pregnancy Loss

Charmila Ayyavoo

■ INTRODUCTION

Recurrent pregnancy loss (RPL) is an important reproductive health issue affecting 2-5% of couples.[1] There are three categories of RPL as primary, secondary, and tertiary RPL. Primary RPL refers to multiple pregnancy losses with no previous viable infants. Secondary RPL refers to multiple losses but with a pregnancy beyond 20 weeks. Tertiary RPL refers to multiple pregnancy losses between normal pregnancies.[2]

Infectious agents are known to cause sporadic pregnancy losses. The organisms implicated in sporadic losses are *Listeria monocytogenes, Toxoplasma gondii,* rubella, herpes simplex virus (HSV), measles, *Cytomegalovirus,* and Coxsackie virus. The incidence of infections causing RPL is proposed to be 0.5-5%.[3,4] The organisms speculated to cause recurrent pregnancy losses are *Mycoplasma, Ureaplasma, Chlamydia trachomatis, Listeria monocytogenes,* and HSV.[5] **Table 1** presents the organisms which probably contribute to recurrent pregnancy losses.[6]

Table 1: Organisms contributing to recurrent pregnancy losses.			
	Bacteria	Viruses	Protozoa
Associated with miscarriage	• Bacterial *vaginosis* (including *Mycoplasma hominis* and *Ureaplasma urealyticum*) • Brucellosis • Syphilis	• Cytomegalovirus • Dengue fever (Flavivirus) • HIV • Rubella	Malaria (Plasmodium)
Little or no evidence for association with miscarriage	*Coxiella burnetii* *Mycoplasma genitalium*	• Adeno-associated virus • Bocavirus • Hepatitis C	None
Conflicting evidence regarding association with miscarriage	*Chlamydia trachomatis*	• Human papillomavirus • Herpes simplex virus 1 and 2 • Parvovirus B19 • Polyomavirus BK • Hepatitis B	*Toxoplasma gondii*

■ PATHOGENESIS

Infections can cause pregnancy losses due to:
- Direct infection of the uterus, fetus or placenta
- Placental insufficiency
- Chronic endometritis (CE) or endocervicitis
- Amnionitis
- Infected intrauterine device.

The above-mentioned mechanisms can cause sporadic losses.[7]

Infections are not commonly associated with RPL. If a patient is susceptible to chronic infection, it may play a role in recurrent fetal losses. The factors which may increase patient susceptibility are:[5]
- Immunocompromised states caused by immune suppressants, chemotherapy, corticosteroids or acquired immune deficiency syndrome.
- The organism's capability to cause an infectious carrier state.
- The capability of the organism to spread to the placenta after the implantation of the embryo.

An infective agent can cause recurrent pregnancy loss if it survives in the genital tract avoiding detection. The knowledge about intrauterine microorganisms is very less compared to the microbes in the vagina. The endometrial cavity is considered to be sterile. But pathogenic microbes have been found in the endometrial cavity without pelvic infection being identified in laparoscopy and negative cervical cultures. In a study by Moller et al. endometrial specimens after hysterectomy were analyzed for microbes. They confirmed the presence of *Gardnerella vaginalis, Enterobacter,* and *Streptococcus agalactiae* in the specimens. The samples were not tested for *Mycoplasma* or *Mobiluncus*.[8]

Except for few studies, there are no confirmed reports of infectious organisms causing RPL. But infections like syphilis, tuberculosis, listeriosis, bacterial vaginosis (BV), *Mycoplasma*, malaria, and *Chlamydia* need a mention in the context of recurrent pregnancy losses.

Chlamydia

There have been conflicting results from the trials conducted on women with habitual miscarriage and chlamydial colonization of the genital tract. In a study by Kishore et al.[9] there was a positive association between positive chlamydia serology and recurrent miscarriage (RM).

Witkin et al. postulated that recurrent pregnancy losses may involve reactivation of latent *Chlamydia* infection, endometrial damage from previous infection or an immune response to an epitope shared by chlamydial and fetal antigens.[10]

Serological testing for chlamydia need not be a part of routine investigation of RPL but a direct swab test from the cervix can be taken. Positive results should be treated with antibiotics.

Syphilis

Pregnancies complicated by untreated syphilis may lead to RPL if it remains untreated in the subsequent pregnancy. The typical history is of recurrent mid-trimester miscarriages with a macerated fetus.[11]

It is also associated with spontaneous abortion, perinatal mortality or a viable infant with congenital syphilis.

Tuberculosis

Genital tuberculosis may cause implantation failure or early embryonic rejection, leading to RPL and ectopic pregnancy.[11]

Listeria and Intracellular Bacteria

Listeria is known to cause sporadic loss. Romana et al.[12] have postulated that latent listeriosis can cause RPL as antilisteric antibodies have been found by direct immune fluorescence studies. In the study of 309 women with RPL, the antilisteric antibodies were identified. Treatment of the infection resulted in the birth of 152 normal babies. Pregnancy loss may be related to the interference with the immune tolerance to the fetus in pregnancy.[13]

Bacterial Vaginosis

Lactobacilli are the predominant organism in the vagina. They metabolize the glycogen in the squamous cells to lactic acid and reduce the pH of the vagina. This provides protection against infection. In BV, there is an overgrowth of anaerobic bacteria and a reduction of lactobacilli. In BV, there is no host reaction. Hence it is named "osis" instead of "itis".[14]

The organisms causing BV are *Gardnerella vaginalis*, group B Streptococci, *Staphylococcus aureus, Ureaplasma urealyticum, Mycoplasma hominis, Mobiluncus* spp., *Prevotella,* Porphyromonas, Bacteroides, and Peptostreptococcus. Bacteroides are gram-negative organisms which are sensitive to metronidazole. *Mycoplasma, Ureaplasma,* and *Mobiluncus* species are sensitive to erythromycin and tetracyclines. They inhabit the endometrial cavity surreptitiously (bacteria endometrialis) and may be responsible for some common gynecological and obstetrical enigmas.[15]

Many studies have proved that BV is associated with premature delivery. Early pregnancy BV is associated with a 2–3-fold increase in premature delivery. Treatment for BV in diagnosed cases has improved the reproductive outcome. If there is a history of previous preterm delivery, BV should be diagnosed and treated. Screening and treatment before pregnancy may be more advantageous.[16]

If not, early second trimester treatment is warranted. BV is less associated with first trimester loss.

Topical antibiotics application in the vagina is less effective than oral antibiotics. This indicates that the microorganisms responsible for preterm labor have ascended out of reach of topical antibiotics and colonized the endometrial cavity. Clindamycin is the antibiotic of choice in BV.[17]

Mycoplasma

Colonization by these organisms in the vagina, cervix has been associated with preterm birth when present in the mid-trimester. The treatment of choice for *Mycoplasma* infections is doxycycline before pregnancy and erythromycin during pregnancy.[18]

■ CHRONIC ENDOMETRITIS

Endometritis can be either acute or chronic. Acute endometritis is characterized by the presence of microabscesses or neutrophils within the endometrial glands, while chronic endometritis is distinguished by variable numbers of plasma cells within the endometrial stroma. Many studies have showed an association of chronic endometritis with RPL (10-27%).[19-21]

Recurrent pregnancy loss is thought to happen in CE due to impaired endometrial receptivity because of:
- Stromal infiltration by plasma cells.
- Alteration in the genes involved in implantation.

Evidence for CE causing RPL has been shown by recent studies. In a study by Inmaculada Moreno et al. in 2016, the presence of endometrial microbes and their impact on implantation have been studied extensively. They examined bacteria from both endometrial fluid and vaginal aspirate samples. They identified different bacterial communities in endometrium and the vagina. The microbes in the endometrial fluid were classified as *Lactobacillus*-dominated microbiota (more than 90% *Lactobacillus* spp.) and a non-*Lactobacillus*-dominated microbiota (NLD) (less than 90% *Lactobacillus* spp. and more than 10% other bacteria). The presence of a non-*Lactobacillus*-dominated microbiota in a receptive endometrium was associated with decreases in implantation rate, pregnancy, ongoing pregnancy, and live birth rates. This demonstrated that pathological modification of bacteria in the endometrium can be associated with poor reproductive outcomes.[22]

Diagnosis

Diagnosis of the disease can be done by hysteroscopy, endometrial biopsy, and identification of plasma cells or microbial culture. The gold standard for diagnosis is the identification of plasma cells in the endometrial stroma by immunohistochemistry stains for syndecan-1 (CD 138) which is a marker of plasma cells.

Newer techniques like real time polymerase chain reaction (PCR) are available to diagnose CE within a short time compared to bacterial cultures which may take a longer time. In a study by Inmaculada et al. in 2018, all the three conventional tests were compared with the molecular diagnostic tool of real time PCR for the presence of 9 chronic endometritis pathogens: *Chlamydia trachomatis, Enterococcus, Escherichia coli, Gardnerella vaginalis, Klebsiella pneumoniae, Mycoplasma hominis, Neisseria gonorrhoeae, Staphylococcus,* and *Streptococcus*. The sensitivity and specificity of the molecular analysis vs. the classic diagnostic techniques were compared in the 65 patients assessed by all three recognized classic methods. More than 50% of the organisms were confirmed by the molecular testing of the microbiology. It also served to diagnose few unculturable organisms in the endometrium. The tests were further confirmed by next generation sequencing of the organisms. In the endometrial samples with concordant histology + hysteroscopy + microbial culture results, the molecular microbiology diagnosis demonstrated 75% sensitivity, 100% specificity, 100% positive and 25% negative predictive values, and 0% false-positive and 25% false-negative rates. The study concluded that molecular microbiology was a rapid and inexpensive tool of diagnosis. It provided detection of culturable and nonculturable microorganisms associated with CE. The concordance rate with all the three classic diagnostic tools was 76.92%. Molecular diagnostic tools were found to be useful in the management of infertile patients who were affected with this ghost endometrial pathology.[23]

Treatment of Chronic Endometritis

The etiology of CE is most probably infectious and favorable outcomes have been reported with antibiotics treatment. Cicinelli et al. evaluated the relationship between RM and CE. The records of 360 women with unexplained RM were retrospectively analyzed. Data from hysteroscopy, endometrial histology, endometrial culture, and polymerase chain reaction (PCR) for *Chlamydia*, performed before and after antibiotic treatment for CE, were analyzed. The occurrence of successful pregnancies within 1 year after treatment was also evaluated. They concluded that CE is frequent in women with RM. Antibiotic treatment seemed to be associated with an improved reproductive outcome.[19]

■ MASSIVE CHRONIC INTERVILLOSITIS

It is a placental disorder which is rare. It has been found to be associated with RPL in the first and second trimester of pregnancy. In later trimester of pregnancy, massive chronic intervillositis (MCI) is found in pregnancies with fetal growth restriction and stillbirths. Studies have associated MCI with maternal infections especially maternal malaria and recurrent sepsis. On histopathological examination, mononuclear cells were identified in the maternal intervillous space and they were sometimes enclosed in fibrin. The intervillous infiltrates were similar to the infiltrates present in chronic villitis of unknown cause. Hence Mariko Horii et al. have also hypothesized an immunologic origin for MCI.[24]

■ TREATMENT IN INFECTIONS AND RECURRENT PREGNANCY LOSS

There are few studies which have postulated that in fertile women the normal uterine microbiome has more than 90% *Lactobacillus*. In the ART population, an altered microbiome that is NLD is associated with lower implantation and higher miscarriage rates.[22]

Presently a clinical trial NCT03401918 is recruiting patients with recurrent pregnancy loss or unexplained infertility to identify whether they have an altered uterine gene expression or uterine microbiome during the window of embryo implantation. They are also assessing whether vaginal progesterone improves gene expression and whether antibiotic treatment followed by probiotic treatment normalizes the microbiome.[25]

■ ANTIBIOTICS IN UNEXPLAINED PREGNANCY LOSSES

In a study by Toth et al. 149 out of 254 couples were treated with antibiotics like doxycycline or tetracycline or erythromycin. All the 254 couples had suffered one or more spontaneous miscarriages. There was a lower incidence of miscarriage in the antibiotic treated group compared to the treated group. The treated group had lesser incidence of premature rupture of membranes, higher vaginal delivery, lower incidence of fetal distress, respiratory distress syndrome, neonatal infection, a higher birth weight, and better Apgar scores.[26]

In a study by Shiffman et al. a group of patients with previous recurrent second trimester losses and failed cervical cerclage were treated with low dose antibiotics till delivery. These patients underwent repeat cerclage at 14–24 weeks of pregnancy along with antibiotic therapy. All the 10 patients achieved fetal viability and their pregnancies were prolonged by a mean of 13.4 + 4.2 weeks beyond their previous pregnancy.[27]

■ CONCLUSION

A disease should be proved to be caused by a specific microorganism based on certain standards which were prescribed by Robert Koch. According to

Koch's postulates, the organism should be isolated from the diseased host and grown in culture. The disease should be reproduced when the cultured material is inoculated in a susceptible host. But these postulates cannot be applied to diseases like syphilis, leprosy, etc. as *Treponema pallidum* and *Mycobacterium leprae* cannot be cultured at all. But the diseases exist. Similarly, the endometrium may be harboring organisms that are resisting cultivation. The development and application of molecular biological techniques in clinical laboratories has made it possible to identify mixed flora including those which could not be grown in culture. Treatment with antibiotics when appropriate will offer solutions to women suffering from recurrent pregnancy losses.

■ REFERENCES

1. Practice Committee of the American Society for Reproductive Medicine. Evaluation and treatment of recurrent pregnancy loss: a committee opinion. Fertility and Sterility. 2012;98(5):1103-11.
2. Kolte AM, Bernardi LA, Christiansen OB, et al. Terminology for pregnancy loss prior to viability: a consensus statement from the ESHRE early pregnancy special interest group. Hum Reprod. 2014;30(3):495-8.
3. Daya S, Stephenson MD. Frequency of factors associated with habitual abortion in 197 couples. Fertil Steril. 1996;66(1):24-9.
4. Fox-Lee L, Schust DJ. Recurrent pregnancy loss. In: Berek JS (Ed). Berek and Novak's Gynecology; 2007. pp. 1277-322.
5. Summers PR. Microbiology relevant to recurrent miscarriage. Clin Obstet Gynecol. 1994;37(3):722-9.
6. Giakoumelou S, Wheelhouse N, Cuschieri K, et al. The role of infection in miscarriage. Hum Reprod Update. 2015;22(1):116-33.
7. Ford HB, Schust DJ. Recurrent pregnancy loss: etiology, diagnosis, and therapy. Rev Obstet Gynecol. 2009;2(2):76.
8. Møller BR, Kristiansen FV, Thorsen P, et al. Sterility of the uterine cavity. Acta obstetricia et gynecologica Scandinavica. 1995;74(3):216-9.
9. Kishore J, Agarwal J, Agrawal S, et al. Seroanalysis of Chlamydia trachomatis and S-TORCH agents in women with recurrent spontaneous abortions. Indian J Pathol Microbiol. 2003;46(4):684-7.
10. Witkin SS, Ledger WJ. Antibodies to Chlamydia trachomatis in sera of women with recurrent spontaneous abortions. Am J Obstet Gynecol. 1992;167(1):135-9.
11. Van Niekerk EC, Siebert I, Kruger TF. An evidence-based approach to recurrent pregnancy loss. S Afr J Obstet Gynaecol. 2013;19(3):61-5.
12. Romana C, Salleras L, Sage M. Latent listeriosis may cause habitual abortion intrauterine deaths, fetal malformations. When diagnosed and treated adequately normal children will be born. Acta Microbiologica Hungarica. 1989;36(2-3):171-2.
13. Rowe JH, Ertelt JM, Way SS. Innate IFN-γ is essential for programmed death ligand-1-mediated T cell stimulation following listeria monocytogenes Infection. J Immunol. 2012;189(2):876-84.

14. Amsel R, Totten PA, Spiegel CA, et al. Nonspecific vaginitis. Diagnostic criteria and microbial and epidemiologic associations. Am J Med. 1983;74(1):14-22.
15. Viniker DA. Hypothesis on the role of sub-clinical bacteria of the endometrium (bacteria endometrialis) in gynaecological and obstetric enigmas. Hum Reprod Update. 1999;5(4):373-85.
16. Rosenstein IJ, Morgan DJ, Lamont RF, et al. Effect of intravaginal clindamycin cream on pregnancy outcome and on abnormal vaginal microbial flora of pregnant women. Infect Dis Obstet Gynecol. 2000;8(3-4):158-65.
17. Lamont RF, Sawant SR. Infection in the prediction and antibiotics in the prevention of spontaneous preterm labour and preterm birth. Minerva Ginecol. 2005;57(4):423-33.
18. Quinn PA, Shewchuk AB, Shuber J, et al. Efficacy of antibiotic therapy in preventing spontaneous pregnancy loss among couples colonized with genital mycoplasmas. Am J Obstet Gynecol. 1983;145(2):239-44.
19. Cicinelli E, Matteo M, Tinelli R, et al. Chronic endometritis due to common bacteria is prevalent in women with recurrent miscarriage as confirmed by improved pregnancy outcome after antibiotic treatment. Reprod Sci. 2014;21(5):640-7.
20. Cicinelli E, Matteo M, Tinelli R, et al. Prevalence of chronic endometritis in repeated unexplained implantation failure and the IVF success rate after antibiotic therapy. Hum Reprod. 2014;30(2):323-30.
21. Valones MA, Guimarães RL, Brandão LA, et al. Principles and applications of polymerase chain reaction in medical diagnostic fields: a review. Braz J Microbiol. 2009;40(1):1-1.
22. Moreno I, Codoñer FM, Vilella F, et al. Evidence that the endometrial microbiota has an effect on implantation success or failure. Am J Obstet Gynecol. 2016;215(6):684-703.
23. Moreno I, Cicinelli E, Garcia-Grau I, et al. The diagnosis of chronic endometritis in infertile asymptomatic women: a comparative study of histology, microbial cultures, hysteroscopy, and molecular microbiology. Am J Obstet Gynecol. 2018;218(6):602-e1.
24. Horii M, Boyd TK, Parast MM. Placental development and complications of previable pregnancy. In: Crum C, Lee K, Nucci M, Granter S, Howitt B, Parast M, Boyd T, Peters III W (Eds). Diagnostic Gynecologic and Obstetric Pathology, 3rd edition. Netherlands: Elsevier; 2017. pp. 1070-102.
25. ClinicalTrials.gov. (2018). Assessing the endometrial environment in recurrent pregnancy loss and unexplained infertility.
26. Toth A, Lesser ML, Brooks-Toth CW, et al. Outcome of subsequent pregnancies following antibiotic therapy after primary or multiple spontaneous abortions. Surg Gynecol Obstet. 1986;163(3):243-50.
27. Shiffman RL. Continuous low-dose antibiotics and cerclage for recurrent second-trimester pregnancy loss. J Reprod Med. 2000;45(4):323-6.

Chapter 13

Preimplantation Genetic Diagnosis: Application and Acceptance in Recurrent Pregnancy Loss

Priya Kannan

■ INTRODUCTION

Human reproduction is a complex process in which there is an extremely complex permutation and combination of the parent genetic material that results in an offspring that has a unique phenotype and genotype, although sharing large parts of genetic material with the parents. Naturally, owing to the complexity of the process, it can have errors. It is estimated that 15–25% of human conceptions fail to reach viability.[1]

■ GENETIC FACTORS IN RECURRENT PREGNANCY LOSS

A vast majority of first trimester pregnancy loss or early pregnancy loss have been attributable to genetic factors. It has been estimated to be as high as 60–70%. The most common factor is chromosomal abnormalities, which could be of parental origin or de novo when the embryo was being formed.[2] By natural selection, 90% of chromosomally abnormal embryos are aborted.

The most common abnormality associated with early pregnancy losses is balanced translocation. Other associated chromosomal abnormalities are Robertsonian translocations, paracentric or pericentric inversions, unbalanced translocations, and aneuploidies such as trisomy, polyploidy, and monosomy X.

Preimplantation Genetic Testing for RPL with Balanced Translocations

A diagnostic modality that would detect the chromosomal abnormality thus significantly reduces the risk of miscarriage and increases the chance of a successful pregnancy is the key to help couples with recurrent pregnancy loss (RPL). Preimplantation genetic testing (PGT) seems to fit the bill perfectly.

Preimplantation genetic testing involves controlled ovarian stimulation, oocyte retrieval, and fertilization of the mature oocytes with sperms of the male partner. The embryos are biopsied and the cells thus got are sent for genetic analysis. The biopsy can be done at the cleavage stage (8 cells) or at the blastocyst stage. When performed at 8-cell stage, one or two blastomeres are specimen for analysis. When done at the blastocyst stage, 5-10 trophectoderm cells are sent the specimen for genetic analysis. The genetic analysis would segregate the normal from the abnormal embryos. The normal embryos are then transferred to the uterus. This process used to be called preimplantation genetic screening (PGS) when a comprehensive screening for all chromosomes is done. When a specific genetic analysis is taken up for a preexistent genetic disorder, such as single gene disorder, it was referred to as preimplantation genetic diagnosis (PGD). However the new terminologies are PGT—PGT-A for aneuploidies, PGT-M for monogenic/single gene defects, and PGT-SR for chromosomal structural rearrangements.

Preimplantation genetic testing has been used as a diagnostic and also as a tool to select the "normal" embryos in cases of RPL secondary to chromosomal abnormalities in parents.

Sugiura-Ogasawara et al. in 2008[3] reported a 63% live birth rate (LBR) with natural conception over a 60-month period. Flynn et al. in 2014[4] reported a cumulative LBR of 64.3% in this group and found no differences in LBR between pregnancies with maternal or paternal carriers as well as those with balanced reciprocal compared with Robertsonian translocations. Franssen et al. published in 2011[5] also demonstrated that 73.5% of couples with RPL and structural chromosome rearrangement achieved a live birth through natural conception, compared with 64-84% cumulative LBR after PGD in a pooled review of case reports.

Fischer et al. in 2012,[6] studied the outcome in 192 patients with RPL with either reciprocal translocation of Robertsonian translocation after PGD and observed a significant decrease in the miscarriage rate (13% vs. 26-64%) and also a significant decrease in the estimated time needed to achieve an ongoing pregnancy (1.4 IVF cycles or 4 months vs. 6 years). The same finding was reiterated by an analysis of data from large studies[7] where PGD was performed for not only couples with RPL but was done for all patients with balanced translocations, the results suggested that miscarriage rates were significantly less in couples who achieved pregnancy following PGT than the general population, though the LBR was ~25-27% per embryo transfer, and ~72% following a positive pregnancy. However two consecutive systematic reviews by the same group found LBR following PGD to be 31-35% compared to 55-74% following natural conception and medical management. Hence, they concluded that there was insufficient data to support PGD in couples with RPL and balanced translocations.

A more recent publication compared pregnancy outcomes in 52 patients with RPL and balanced translocations who had natural conception and 37 matched patients who opted for PGD using fluorescence in situ hybridization

(FISH) analysis.[8] The study found no differences in the LBR at the first trial (37.8% vs. 53.8%, respectively), in the cumulative LBR (67.6% vs. 65.4%, respectively), and in the mean interval of months from genetic counseling to the pregnancy (12.4 vs. 11.4, respectively). However, PGD significantly decreased the mean number of miscarriages (0.22 ± 0.42 vs. 0.58 ± 0.78, P = 0.012) and significantly increased the number of twin pregnancies. Another study[9] in 2016 reported a similar LBR and miscarriage rate in patients who did or did not undergo PGD but also found no reduction in miscarriage with PGD. In a retrospective cohort study[10] of 300 RPL patients, clinical pregnancy rate per euploid embryo transfer was 72% and LB rate per euploid embryo transfer was 57%. Among all attempts at preimplantation genetic screening (PGS) or expectant management, clinical outcomes were similar. Median time to pregnancy was 6.5 months in the PGS group and 3.0 months in the EM group.

Hence, current evidence suggests that good reproductive outcomes can be achieved through expectant management among patients who are evaluated and treated for other reversible causes of RPL. There was insufficient data to support systematic PGD in couples with RPL and balanced translocations.[11] The concept that PGT-A in patients with RPL and balanced translocation reduces miscarriage rate should also be studied more. However, the advantage of PGT-A should be weighed against the procedure of PGT which is expensive and does not guarantee creation normal embryos or pregnancy. COI and PGT in itself cause huge emotional stress and burden.

Preimplantation Genetic Testing for Unexplained RPL

Preimplantation genetic screening or present day PGT-A, has been proposed as an option for couples with unexplained recurrent pregnancy loss (URPL). In a landmark paper, Santiago Munne and his colleagues demonstrated the high percentage of aneuploidy in embryos in assisted reproductive technology (ART).[12] Hence PGS was first introduced in 1993 to select euploid embryos in infertile couples undergoing IVF, thus hoping to transfer the embryos with the highest developmental potential, which would result in improving implantation rates and decreasing miscarriage rates.

PGT-A should ideally involve the analysis of all 23 chromosome pairs. Many techniques have been used over the years, namely FISH, comparative genome hybridization (CGH), array CGH (aCGH), single nucleotide polymorphism array, quantitative or real-time polymerase chain reaction, and next-generation sequencing (NGS) also known as massive parallel sequencing. FISH was the first technique to be used where only a few chromosomes could be studied. However, studies failed to show any advantage of doing PGT-A using FISH and on the other hand some publications showed that it could actually be deleterious.[13] Inabilities to screen all chromosomes, embryo mosaicism, and cleavage stage biopsy were the main reasons for the failure of FISH as technique for PGS. Presently the newer techniques allow for screening of all chromosomes and the trophectoderm biopsy has become the norm, where the mosaicism is significantly much lesser (3–5%). All the molecular techniques presently applied in PGT-A are not equally efficient, and although they can all detect whole chromosome aneuploidy, they differ in their abilities to identify mosaicism, as well as other structural abnormalities, and their lowest detection thresholds.[14]

A recent meta-analysis[15] concluded that the transfer of euploid embryos following PGS significantly improves pregnancy rates. However, the randomized controlled trials (RCTs) included in the meta-analysis had studied young patients with normal ovarian reserve and good prognosis, and hence extrapolating these results to other patient population is unfair. Indeed, no RCTs have looked at the beneficial impact of PGS in couples with RPL and normal karyotypes.

The conclusion of the authors of the Cochrane study with the research question, preimplantation genetic screening (PGS) for abnormal number of chromosomes in assisted reproduction, reads—"PGS as currently performed significantly decreases live birth rates in women of advanced maternal age and those with repeated IVF failure. Trials in which PGS was offered to women with a good prognosis suggested similar outcomes. PGS technique development is still ongoing in an effort to increase its efficacy. This involves biopsy at other stages of development (polar body or trophectoderm biopsy) and other methods of analysis [comparative genome hybridization (CGH) or array-based technologies] than used by the trials included in this review. These new developments should be properly evaluated before their routine clinical application. Until such trials have been performed, PGS should not be offered as routine patient care in any form".

■ CONCLUSION

As per the present published evidence, PGT-A for patients with RPL has no established advantage over spontaneous conception with expectant management.

■ ACCEPTANCE AMONG PROFESSIONALS

A survey of 30 participants was conducted with questions specific to PGS 2.0. A questionnaire was developed on the three major aspects of PGS 2.0: the Why, with general questions such as PGS 2.0 indications; the How, specifically on genetic analysis methods; the When, on the ideal method and timing of embryo biopsy.[16]

The 30 participants were mainly from Europe (Belgium, Germany, Greece, Italy, Netherlands, Spain, UK) and the USA. The result of the questionnaire is as below.

The most common technique of analysis used by the participants was array comparative genome hybridization 9aCGH and most were in the process of switching to NGS as the method of choice of analysis.

Blastocyst was the most preferred stage for biopsy.

There is varying opinions on offering PGS 2.0 to all patients. Some were more inclined to offer PGS 2.0 to all patients, were also using the technique for selection of embryos, while some were skeptical on routine use of PGS, and rather preferring to wait for more reliable date on the reliability of the technique.

■ REFERENCES

1. El Hachem H, Crepaux V, May-Panloup P, et al. Recurrent pregnancy loss: current perspectives. Int J Womens Health. 2017;9:331-45.
2. Sugiura-Ogasawara M, Ozaki Y, Katano K, et al. Abnormal embryonic karyotype is the most frequent cause of recurrent miscarriage. Hum Reprod. 2012;27(8):2297-303.
3. Sugiura-Ogasawara M, Aoki K, Fujii T, et al. Subsequent pregnancy outcomes in recurrent miscarriage patients with a paternal or maternal carrier of a structural chromosome rearrangement. J Hum Genet. 2008;53:622-8.
4. Flynn H, Yan J, Saravelos SH, et al. Comparison of reproductive outcome, including the pattern of loss, between couples with chromosomal abnormalities and those with unexplained repeated miscarriages. J Obstet Gynaecol Res. 2014;40:109-16.
5. Franssen MT, Musters AM, van der Veen F, et al. Reproductive outcome after PGD in couples with recurrent miscarriage carrying a structural chromosome abnormality: a systematic review. Hum Reprod Update. 2011;17(4):467-75.
6. Fischer J, Colls P, Escudero T, et al. Preimplantation genetic diagnosis (PGD) improves pregnancy outcome for translocation carriers with a history of recurrent losses. Fertil Steril. 2010;94(1):283-9.
7. De Rycke M, Belva F, Goossens V, et al. ESHRE PGD Consortium data collection XIII: cycles from January to December 2010 with pregnancy follow-up to October 2011. Hum Reprod. 2015;30(8):1763-89.
8. Ikuma S, Sato T, Sugiura-Ogasawara M, et al. Preimplantation genetic diagnosis and natural conception: a comparison of live birth rates in patients with recurrent pregnancy loss associated with translocation. PLoS ONE. 2015;10(6):e0129958.
9. Bedaiwy M, Maithripala S, Durland U, et al. Reproductive outcomes of couples with recurrent pregnancy loss due to parental chromosome rearrangement. Fertil Steril. 2016;106:e343.
10. Murugappan G, Shahine LK, Perfetto CO, et al. Intent to treat analysis of in vitro fertilization and preimplantation genetic screening versus expectant management in patients with recurrent pregnancy loss. Hum Reprod. 2016; 31(8):1668-74.

11. Iews M, Tan J, Taskin O, Alfaraj S, et al. Does preimplantation genetic diagnosis improve reproductive outcome in couples with recurrent pregnancy loss owing to structural chromosomal rearrangement? A systematic review. Reprod Biomed Online. 2018;36(6):677-85.
12. Munne S, Lee A, Rosenwaks Z, et al. Diagnosis of major chromosome aneuploidies in human preimplantation embryos. Hum Reprod. 1993;8(12):2185-91.
13. Mastenbroek S, Twisk M, van der Veen F, et al. Preimplantation genetic screening: a systematic review and meta-analysis of RCTs. Hum Reprod Update. 2011;17(4):454-66.
14. Geraedts J, Sermon K. Preimplantation genetic screening 2.0: the theory. Mol Hum Reprod. 2016;22(8):839-44.
15. Dahdouh EM, Balayla J, García-Velasco JA. Comprehensive chromosome screening improves embryo selection: a meta-analysis. Fertil Steril. 2015;104(6):1503-12.
16. Sermon K, Capalbo A, Cohen J, et al. The why, the how and the when of PGS 2.0: current practices and expert opinions of fertility specialists, molecular biologists, and embryologists. Mol Hum Reprod. 2016;22(8):545-57.

Chapter 14: Setting up a Recurrent Pregnancy Loss Clinic

Suchitra N Pandit, Ashwini Ingale

■ INTRODUCTION

A clinic with outpatient specialist services for couples suffering from recurrent pregnancy losses (RPL) should be set up if possible as a part of obstetric services. It should offer the entire basket of services like investigation of the couple, psychological counseling, a support system, and management services for all conditions.

Providing details and data about RPL to the suffering couple should be an important goal of the clinic. The couple should be informed with no ambiguity that even if extensively investigated, there may be very less management options available at the end.

■ ACCESS TO CARE

When couples have undergone repeated pregnancy losses which may be two or more, they need to be referred to the clinics which offer special services and are headed by consultants trained in managing RPL. The specialist services should be focused and devoted to managing RPL. These clinics should not be part of emergency services. The couples should be encouraged to attend these clinics and undergo the necessary investigations and formulate a management strategy. This is an absolute necessity before the next pregnancy.

■ THE RECURRENT PREGNANCY LOSS CLINIC

There are prerequisites for a clinic specializing in RPL services. They are discussed next.[1]

Personnel Needed

The members of the team managing this emotionally sensitive problem should be well trained in all aspects of care of RPL. They include specialists in reproductive medicine, nurses trained in these aspects of healthcare, obstetricians, and gynecologists. There should be specialists trained in ultrasonography in the team. The group should have special skills for listening to the couples and manage them with sympathy and empathy.

First Visit

The visit of the couples to the RPL clinic for the first time is the most crucial visit. When the couple's appointment is fixed, details about what is awaiting them during the consultation should be offered. This would help to reduce anxiety in the couple. During the first visit, adequate time should be spent by the specialist in analyzing the couple's history and providing replies to them. An algorithm for the proposed investigations should be prepared. A management strategy should be formulated at the initial visit.

Location

The outpatient clinic is preferably located in a quiet area away from the antenatal clinic, pediatric clinic, maternity unit or obstetrics department ward. Area should be calm, well-lit, and have pleasant décor. Facilities should include a clean toilet, drinking water, and counter for tea/coffee.

Equipment

The clinic should have excellent appropriate imaging facilities which include ultrasound provision and 3D ultrasound. The clinic should also have a tie-up with the required laboratories so that the necessary investigations can be done with accuracy.

Dissemination of Knowledge

During the initial visit itself, the couple should be provided details about the reasons for RPL, the frequency of the condition, and the management options. Efforts should be made to provide particulars based on the couple's history. The couple should be given enough time to articulate their questions and doubts to the specialists during the initial and later visits. The specialist should refrain from using their cell phones during the couples visit.

The members of the RPL clinic should know that most of the couples coming for a consultation would have already accrued knowledge about the condition. They would be asking for clarifications and their information would need some renewal. Facilities should be available to provide pamphlets from other sources like accepted guidelines of reputed societies, professional bodies to the couple. Special meetings where they can meet with other couples suffering from the same condition can be offered. These meetings can be utilized to impart information to the couples.

Assessment of the Couple

The patient and her husband should be questioned thoroughly on menstrual history, marital history, obstetric history, past medical history, surgical history, family history, and all the tests they have undergone in the past. The treatments they have undergone should also be extensively asked for. As a part of the consultation, the perspective of the couple regarding the tests and management plan should be solicited.

It is imperative that the couple understands before undergoing any test that it may not diagnose a reason for RPL. They should also be counseled regarding the fact there may be conditions which even after diagnosis do not have management options. They should understand that even if treatments are available, they can be unpredictable.

Information regarding time span for the required tests and the scrutiny of outcomes should be shared with the couple. The couples may have queries on the need for postponing their next pregnancy while they are waiting for the results.

Customized Psychological Counseling

The staff member providing counseling to the bereaved couple needs to be attuned to their needs. Adequate time should be spent in history taking and all details pertaining to their case should be discussed. This type of empathetic dialogue would provide a great support to the couple. The counselor should listen to all their grievances and should take into count the couple's emotions and experiences. The vocabulary used in the sessions with the couple should be tactful and thoughtful.

Planning and Approach

The couples suffering from RPL come with the preconceived idea that the tests that they undergo to diagnose the cause would also lead to a management plan which would prove successful. If the tests do not show a recognized cause for their loss, they could become distraught. This could happen even if data show that the prognosis is good for many couples. An additional backup plan should be devised for such couples in their next pregnancy so that they undergo a planned antenatal checkup. They could be counseled to participate in clinical trials too. If a cause for the RPL is identified but the management has no confirmed outcomes, the couple should be provided with more educational material about the pros and cons of the management protocol.

Research

Couples suffering from RPL are very sensitive and they should not be offered treatments which are done for the purpose of research. They are unguarded and may subject themselves to treatments which have a chance of giving them a successful outcome. Some patients are more open to new management protocols and would be willing to participate in some type of qualitative research or in clinical trials. They may feel that they are participating in productive work for themselves as well as for the community. The staff members can provide information about these methods to the couple during a regular visit. Deliberations on the methods should be conducted in other meetings with the couple.

■ MANAGEMENT STRATEGY

The strategy for management of couples suffering from RPL should be formulated for their medical therapy, psychological aid, and supportive care. Patients visiting a specialist clinic for RPL come expecting a diagnosis of the cause and an accepted management protocol for the condition which would prevent future losses in pregnancy. Many of them would have undergone checkups with other specialists and would have already accrued information about their problem.

The management strategy of such couples entails future plans in their medications and changes in their lifestyle whenever needed. An important part of the discussion should be on their preference for a particular consultant, the timing of scans, and consultations. The staff members of the entire team should have the aptitude of showing attention to the troubles of the couple, a thorough understanding of the obstetric history, empathy, and consideration for the couple's pain.

The management options for each couple are different and this has to be borne in mind during treatment. The emotional condition and needs of each patient is different. Hence a solitary model of treatment cannot be advised for all couples. The following points should be kept in mind when formulating a plan for the patient. The staff members of the RPL clinic should be readily available and they should have undergone rigorous training for the job. They should be capable of providing care which is needed for the couple and should be attuned to the couple's needs. The important staff members who form the support system of the RPL clinic are counselors, psychologists, and social workers. The following points should be kept in mind during the management of this delicate issue:

- Acknowledgement of the patient as a separate entity: she, her partner, her history, her baby, this instance.
- Adequate hours spent on queries, details, doubts, and treatment plans. If the patient is anguished, more time should be spent with her.
- Establish a good rapport with the couple and listen to their emotional needs.
- Deference should be shown to the woman, her partner, the children she has lost, and for her anxieties and choices. Her ideas may not be viable but they should be listened to with care.

- The word used to express the treatment options should be attuned to the couple's needs. It should be concise, precise, and words like recurrent aborter, products of conception, blighted ovum, incompetent cervix, and pregnancy failure should not be used. The conversation with the couple should have a positive connotation like baby, pregnancy, etc.
- Truthful facts about the treatments, results, and prognosis should be provided. Dishonest commiserations should not be done.
- The method of dispersing details so that the couple has a feeling of participating in the entire process would give a sense of control to the couple.
- The subsequent pregnancy should be managed by providing care both in person and through telephones regarding their visits, the tests needed and the dates of their scan. These couples should be given priority in care.
- The care shown to the couple should be filled with warmth and generosity.
- Provision of a telephone number for any queries is essential.
- Feedback forms and information about successful pregnancy outcomes should be displayed on the board so it gives encouragement to the distressed couples.

■ CONCLUSION

"Selfishness is a weakness. But loving and caring for others is a position of power beyond anything we can possibly imagine" is a quote by Joel Osteen. Providing the services for a comprehensive evaluation of all factors which can contribute to pregnancy loss is a must for a team involved in management of couples who have suffered repeated pregnancy losses. It is equally important that the emotional needs of the couple are also taken care of by the service provider. Setting up a RPL clinic for these purposes by clinicians in a position of power to help the distressed couples is a service to society.

■ REFERENCE

1. ESHRE Guideline Group on RPL, Bender Atik R, Christiansen OB, Elson J, Kolte AM, Lewis S, Middeldorp S, Nelen W, Peramo B, Quenby S, Vermeulen N. ESHRE guideline: recurrent pregnancy loss.

Chapter 15: Role of Assisted Reproduction in Recurrent Pregnancy Loss

Nandita Palshetkar, Manisha T Kundnani

■ INTRODUCTION

Recurrent pregnancy loss (RPL) is a distressing situation for the couple and a frustrating problem for the treating clinician as many times in spite of thorough workup no cause is identified. This leaves the couples anxious and full of uncertainty about the future pregnancies. Of all the known causes of recurrent abortions (namely uterine anomalies, autoimmune disorders, thrombophilias, metabolic and hormonal disorders, chronic endometritis), embryo aneuploidy or other chromosomal defects in the embryo are the most common causes of first trimester recurrent miscarriage. In vitro fertilization (IVF) along with preimplantation genetic screening (PGS) can help select normal euploid embryos for transfer and can thus increase the live birth rates in patients with balanced chromosomal translocations or unexplained RPL.

■ CYTOGENETIC ABNORMALITY AND RECURRENT PREGNANCY LOSS

A large proportion of early pregnancy losses is attributed to chromosomal abnormalities, which can either arise de novo or can be of parental origin.[1,2] It has been observed that collectively parental and embryonic factors can provide an explanation in most couples (~90%) with recurrent miscarriages.[3]

Embryonic aneuploidies (trisomy, monosomy, polyploidy, and other chromosomal errors) are the most common cause of early trimester pregnancy loss. The importance of embryonic aneuploidy is highlighted by the fact that approximately 40–50% of these miscarriages are chromosomally abnormal and the risk increases with maternal age.[4] It has been observed that meiotic chromosome segregation errors increase with the increasing age.[5] Such meiotic errors can either result in an extra chromosome (trisomy) or deletion of a chromosome (monosomy). Fertilization of an oocyte by two spermatozoa can lead to triploidy (complete set of extra chromosomes), or failure of completion of first zygotic division can cause tetraploidy. Some of these couples are at risk of recurrent aneuploidy involving different chromosomes (heterotrisomy).[6]

However, as most cases occur de novo, the chances of aneuploidy conceptus in the future pregnancies is low and unpredictable. So, as the number of miscarriages increase, it is unlikely that it is because of chromosomal abnormalities. Karyotyping products of conception helps in clinical investigation and can help predict outcome of subsequent pregnancies. Women who miscarry a euploid (normal chromosome complement) embryo have a greater risk of recurrent miscarriages than women who lost aneuploidy pregnancy.[7]

Balanced translocations are the most common parental abnormality found in patients with RPL. The incidence is 2-4% in couples with RPL compared to 0.7% in general population. These translocations can be reciprocal (~60%) or Robertsonian (~40%). Paracentric and pericentric inversions are also associated with enhanced risk of RPL.[8,9] These defects can be identified on parental karyotyping.

The carriers of balanced translocation are usually asymptomatic, but their conceptus can either be normal or may carry a balanced or unbalanced translocation. Those with unbalanced translocations usually result in a miscarriage, or still births or live births with major congenital anomalies. It has been observed that approximately 25-40% of miscarried fetuses have unbalanced translocations.[10,11] However, in spite of the increased risk of miscarriage, many couples with balanced translocations usually have healthy babies.[10] These patients should be referred to a clinical geneticist and thoroughly counseled about the chances of repeat abortions and successful pregnancies.

■ MALE CONTRIBUTION TO RECURRENT PREGNANCY LOSS

Male contribution to RPL was mostly unexplored till recently and was limited to paternal karyotype as most of these patients had normal semen parameters. However, male factors which can contribute to recurrent pregnancy losses have been studied recently and several factors like sperm motility, morphological sperm alterations, sperm DNA fragmentation, and sperm aneuploidy have been found to be associated with RPL.[12,13]

DNA Fragmentation and RPL

Sperm integrity is of vital importance for initiation and maintenance of successful pregnancy, and fertilization of an oocyte with damaged sperms can lead to damaged embryo genome which can cause DNA errors at various stages of embryogenesis. Many studies have suggested an association between increased sperm DNA fragmentation and recurrent pregnancy loss.[14-18] Abnormal packaging of sperm chromatin causes increased DNA fragmentation and can be seen in males with advanced age or with exogenous factors that increase oxidative stress like varicocele, smoking, exogenous heat, and occupational exposure to toxins.

Bareh et al. reported significantly high sperm DNA fragmentation in couples with RPL compared to control group. Interestingly males in both groups were normozoospermic.[19] As the paternal genome is activated between the 4- and 8-cell stage in human embryos, it has been suggested that high DNA damage may have no effect on initial fertilization but can manifest in later stages of embryonic development.[20,21]

Various interventions have been proposed to decrease sperm DNA fragmentation. The males should be advised to avoid all exogenous factors (smoking, alcohol, environmental toxins) that can increase DNA fragmentation. Varicoceles are a known cause of sperm DNA damage and varicocelectomy has been found beneficial in many such patients.[22,23] A randomized controlled trial (RCT) conducted by Mansour et al. demonstrated higher conception and lower miscarriage rates after varicocele surgery in couples with RPL.[24] In severe cases, intracytoplasmic sperm injection (ICSI) with testicular sperms has been shown to have better outcomes compared to ejaculated sperms.[25] Sperm donation is another option in case of very high DNA fragmentation index (DFI).

However, despite many studies showing possible etiological role of DNA fragmentation in RPL, its use is limited as the cut-off of abnormal high DFI varies in different studies and measurement methodology still needs to be standardized.

Sperm Aneuploidy and RPL

Sperm aneuploidy is another male parameter that has recently been investigated as a potential cause of RPL. The causes of sperm aneuploidy can be nondisjunction, anaphase lag, or inefficient checkpoint control. Ramasamy et al. observed that up to 40% of men with RPL have aneuploid sperms.[26] A high rate of disomy, diploidy, sex chromosome disomy, nullisomy, and total aneuploidy is observed in the sperms from these patients. In a recent study conducted by Neusser et al., increased aneuploidy for chromosomes 16, 2, 1, 21, 4, and 6 was observed in male partners with RPL.[27] Selection of euploid sperm for fertilization could possibly improve the chances of successful pregnancy in these couples, however, no such technique is yet available. IVF with PGS seems a viable treatment option in such patients.

■ PREIMPLANTATION GENETIC DIAGNOSIS AND PREIMPLANTATION GENETIC SCREENING FOR RECURRENT PREGNANCY LOSS

As cytogenetic abnormalities in the embryo, including inherited unbalanced translocations and de novo aneuploidy, are responsible for a significant number of recurrent pregnancy losses, selecting only chromosomally normal embryos for transfer, and screening out aneuploidies via IVF–PGS has been utilized as a management option for couples with unexplained RPL and in carriers of balanced translocations. It requires the couple to undergo IVF to produce embryos which are and then biopsied, analyzed, and frozen; and normal embryos are then transferred in subsequent cycles.

Embryos can be tested by preimplantation genetic diagnosis (PGD) for specific genetic abnormalities which are heritable or present in either of the partners; or PGS which is a more global genetic assessment and is more commonly used in patients with idiopathic RPL.

Various techniques including fluorescent in situ hybridization (FISH), comparative genomic hybridization (CGH), single-nucleotide polymorphism (SNP) array, polymerase chain reaction (PCR), and next-generation sequencing (NGS) have been utilized for PGS. FISH was the first technique utilized for PGS. However, earlier studies with IVF–FISH failed to show any beneficial effect as only limited number of chromosomes could be analyzed with this technique.[28,29] Also, the chances of mosaicism are high on day 3 embryos, so the biopsied cell may not be representative of the whole embryo. The newer techniques like CGH and NGS involve whole genome sequencing. Also, the embryos are biopsied at blastocyst stage where the chances of mosaicism and damage to the embryo are significantly low, and all 23 pairs of chromosomes are analyzed.[30,31]

PGD in Carriers of Balanced Translocation

Preimplantation genetic screening seems to be a rational choice in the case of parental chromosomal translocations and recurrent miscarriages. It has been shown that it can decrease the miscarriage rate from 88.5% to 13% in translocation carriers.[32] However, if the couple is unwilling for IVF, chorionic villous sampling or amniocentesis during pregnancy are the other options available. Oocyte or sperm donation can be the last resort in some of these couples.

PGS for Unexplained RPL

Though it has been shown that transfer of euploid embryos after PGS significantly increases live birth rates in infertile women with normal ovarian reserve and good prognosis,[33-35] it is difficult to extrapolate the same data to women with unexplained RPL. There is scarcity of data proving the efficacy of IVF–PGS over expectant management in patients with RPL. No prospective studies or well powered randomized clinical trials have yet been performed in this area. The available data is mostly retrospective and with several limitations. The cost of the procedure and the live birth rate per initiated PGS cycles should be kept in mind before offering this treatment to couples with unexplained RPL.

A cost-effective analysis conducted by Murugappan et al. comparing IVF-PGS vs. expectant management found that live birth rate was similar in both groups and IVF-PGS was 100 times more expensive than expectant management.[36] Studies that identify which patients are most likely to benefit from PGS and include live birth rates per initiated cycles are needed before universally recommending this treatment to couples with RPL.

ROLE OF SURROGACY IN RECURRENT PREGNANCY LOSS

Surrogacy for couples with RPL works on the principle that the embryo is normal and that the maternal environment needs to be changed. It has been suggested that as the number of miscarriages increases the likelihood of chromosomal aberrations being the cause decreases, and so these patients may get benefitted by changing uterine environment. Many authors have reported successful live births by surrogacy after multiple recurrent losses (as high as up to 24 losses).[37] Women losing euploid embryos can be advised to consider surrogacy.

Some patients with autoimmune conditions and recurrent abortions, including the antiphospholipid antibody syndrome (APS), who show no improvement despite anticoagulants and aspirin, can also be candidates for surrogacy.

Unfortunately, surrogacy as an effective treatment modality has limited application, as it is banned in many countries and there are stringent guidelines and laws governing it in many other countries.

CONCLUSION

The "seed" which is the embryo or the "soil" which is the endometrium may be the reason for recurrent pregnancy losses in a couple. Analyzing the embryo with PGS before transfer or changing the endometrium with surrogacy in ART has not be proven to be of benefit. More advancements in ART technologies are needed before assisted reproduction can be offered as a solution in the treatment of recurrent pregnancy losses.

REFERENCES

1. Sugiura-Ogasawara M, Ozaki Y, Katano K, et al. Abnormal embryonic karyotype is the most frequent cause of recurrent miscarriage. Hum Reprod. 2012;27: 2297-303.
2. Werner M, Reh A, Grifo J, et al. Characteristics of chromosomal abnormalities diagnosed after spontaneous abortions in an infertile population. J Assist Reprod Genet. 2012;29:817-20.

3. Popescu F, Jaslow CR, Kutteh WH. Recurrent pregnancy loss evaluation combined with 24 chromosome micro array of miscarriage tissue provides a probable or definite cause of pregnancy loss in over 90% of patients. Hum Reprod. 2018;33:579-87.
4. Zhang T, Sun Y, Chen Z, et al. Traditional and molecular chromosomal abnormality analysis of products of conception in spontaneous and recurrent miscarriages. BJOG. 2018;125:414-20.
5. Greaney J, Wei Z, Homer H. Regulation of chromosome segregation in oocytes and the cellular basis for female meiotic errors. Hum Reprod Update. 2018;24:135-61.
6. Warburton D, Dallaire L, Thangavelu M, et al. Trisomy recurrence: a reconsideration based on North American data. Am J Hum Genet. 2004;75:376-85.
7. Ogasawara M, Aoki K, Okada S, et al. Embryonic karyotype of abortuses in relation to the number of previous miscarriages. Fertil Steril. 2000;73:300-4.
8. De Braekeleer M, Dao TN. Cytogenetic studies in couples experiencing recurrent pregnancy loss. Hum Reprod. 1990;5:519-28.
9. Laurino MY, Bennett RL, Saraiya DS, et al. Genetic evaluation and counselling of couples with recurrent miscarriages: recommendations of the National Society of Genetic Counselors. J Genet Couns. 2005;14:165-81.
10. Stephenson MD, Sierra S. Reproductive outcomes in recurrent pregnancy loss associated with a parental carrier of structural chromosome rearrangement. Hum Reprod. 2006;21:1076-82.
11. Carp H, Guetta E, Dorf H, et al. Embryonic karyotype in recurrent miscarriage with parental karyotypic aberrations. Fertil Steril. 2006;85:446-50.
12. Bhattacharya SM. Association of various sperm parameters with unexplained repeated early pregnancy loss—which is most important? Int Urol Nephrol. 2008;40:391-5.
13. Bernardini LM, Costa M, Bottazzi C, et al. Sperm aneuploidy and recurrent pregnancy loss. Reprod BioMed Online. 2004;9:312-20.
14. Saxena P, Misro MM, Chaki SP, et al. Is abnormal sperm function an indicator among couples with recurrent pregnancy loss? Fertil Steril. 2008;90:1854-8.
15. Brahem S, Mehdi M, Landolsi H, et al. Semen parameters and sperm DNA fragmentation as causes of recurrent pregnancy loss. Urology. 2011;78:792-6.
16. Zidi-Jrah I, Hajlaoui A, Mougou-Zerelli S, et al. Relationship between sperm aneuploidy, sperm DNA integrity, chromatin packaging, traditional semen parameters, and recurrent pregnancy loss. Fertil Steril. 2016;105:58-64.
17. Gil-Villa AM, Cardona-Maya W, Agarwal A, et al. Assessment of sperm factors possibly involved in early recurrent pregnancy loss. Fertil Steril. 2010;94:1465-72.
18. Khadem N, Poorhoseyni A, Jalali M, et al. Sperm DNA fragmentation in couples with unexplained recurrent spontaneous abortions. Andrologia. 2014;46:126-30.
19. Bareh GM, Jacoby E, Binkley P, et al. Sperm deoxyribonucleic acid fragmentation assessment in normozoospermic male partners of couples with unexplained recurrent pregnancy loss: a prospective study. Fertil Steril. 2016;105:329-36.
20. Virro MR, Larson-Cook KL, Evenson DP. Sperm chromatin structure assay (SCSA) parameters are related to fertilization, blastocyst development, and ongoing pregnancy in in vitro fertilization and intracytoplasmic sperm injection cycles. Fertil Steril. 2004;81:1289-95.
21. Braude P, Bolton V, Moore S. Human gene expression first occurs between the four- and eight-cell stages of preimplantation development. Nature. 1988;332:459-61.

22. Wang YJ, Zhang RQ, Lin YJ, et al. Relationship between varicocele and sperm DNA damage and the effect of varicocele repair: a meta-analysis. Reprod Biomed Online. 2012;25:307-14.
23. Kadioglu TC, Aliyev E, Celtik M. Microscopic varicocelectomy significantly decreases the sperm DNA fragmentation index in patients with infertility. Biomed Res Int. 2014; 2014:695713.
24. Mansour Ghanaie M, Asgari SA, Dadrass N, et al. Effects of varicocele repair on spontaneous first trimester miscarriage: a randomized clinical trial. Urol J. 2012;9:505-13.
25. Esteves SC, Sánchez-Martín F, Sánchez-Martín P, et al. Comparison of reproductive outcome in oligozoospermic men with high sperm DNA fragmentation undergoing intracytoplasmic sperm injection with ejaculated and testicular sperm. Fertil Steril. 2015;104:1398-405.
26. Ramasamy R, Scovell JM, Kovac JR, et al. Fluorescence in situ hybridization detects increased sperm aneuploidy in men with recurrent pregnancy loss. Fertil Steril. 2015;103:906-9.
27. Neusser M, Rogenhofer N, Durl S, et al. Increased chromosome 16 disomy rates in human spermatozoa and recurrent spontaneous abortions. Fertil Steril. 2015;104:1130-7.
28. Munne S, Lee A, Rosenwaks Z, et al. Diagnosis of major chromosome aneuploidies in human preimplantation embryos. Hum Reprod. 1993;8: 2185-91.
29. Mastenbroek S, Twisk M, van der Veen F, et al. Preimplantation genetic screening: a systematic review and meta-analysis of RCT's. Hum Reprod Update. 2011;17:454-66.
30. Scott RT, Upham KM, Forman EJ, et al. Cleavage stage biopsy significantly impairs human embryonic implantation potential while blastocyst biopsy does not: a randomised and paired clinical trial. Fertil Steril. 2013;100:624-30.
31. Brezina PR, Anchan R, Kearns WG. Preimplantation genetic testing for aneuploidy: what technology should you use and what are the differences? J Assist Reprod Genet. 2016;33:823-32.
32. Ikuma S, Sato T, Sugiura-Ogasawara M, et al. Preimplantation genetic diagnosis and natural conception: a comparison of live birth rates in patients with recurrent pregnancy loss associated with translocation. PLoS ONE. 2015;10(6):e0129958.
33. Yang Z, Liu J, Collins GS, et al. Selection of single blastocysts for fresh transfer via standard morphology assessment alone and with array CGH for good prognosis IVF patients: results from randomised pilot study. Mol Cytogenet. 2012;5:24.
34. Forman EJ, Hong KH, Ferry KM, et al. In vitro fertilisation with single euploid blastocyst transfer: a randomised controlled trial. Fertil Steril. 2013;100:100-7.
35. Scott RT Jr, Upham KM, Forman EJ, et al. Blastocyst biopsy with comprehensive chromosome screening and fresh embryo transfer significantly increases in vitro fertilisation implantation and delivery rates: a randomised controlled trial. Fertil Steril. 2013;100:697-703.
36. Murugappan G, Ohno MS, Lathi RB. Cost-effectiveness analysis of preimplantation genetic screening and in vitro fertilization versus expectant management in patients with unexplained recurrent pregnancy loss. Fertil Steril. 2015;103(5):1215-20.
37. Carp HJA, Dirnfeld M, Dor J, et al. ART in recurrent miscarriage: preimplantation genetic diagnosis/screening or surrogacy? Hum Reprod. 2004;19:1502-5.

Chapter 16: Immunotherapy in Recurrent Pregnancy Loss

Hrishikesh D Pai, Manisha T Kundnani

■ INTRODUCTION

Approximately 1–2% of couples are affected by recurrent pregnancy loss and this causes a significant physical, emotional and psychological burden on them. A number of therapies have been implemented over the years based on the various known causes of recurrent abortions. Cytogenetic abnormalities, uterine anomalies, antiphospholipid antibody syndrome, hormonal and metabolic disorders, inherited thrombophilias, chronic endometritis and luteal phase defect are the commonly established causes of RPL.[1] However, in more than 50% of couples there are no discernible causes. It has been suggested that immune dysregulation can be the cause of fetal rejection and pregnancy loss in many such patients. It has also been observed that with the increase in the number of miscarriages, the likelihood of alloimmunity or immunological aberrations increases.[2] Immunomodulatory therapies like paternal leucocyte immunization (LIT), intravenous immunoglobulin (IVIG), intralipids, trophoblastic infusions, third party donor cell immunizations anti TNF-α drugs and granulocyte colony stimulating factor (G-CSF) have been used in such patients with controversial results.

■ MATERNOFETAL ALLOIMMUNE RESPONSE

A successful pregnancy depends on maternal immunologic tolerance of the semiallogenic fetus, as allogenic paternal human leukocyte antigens (HLAs) are presented to the maternal immune system. For healthy implantation and pregnancy, maternal immune system should allow as well as restrict fetal cytotrophoblastic invasion. A bidirectional communication regulated by various maternal immune mediator cells, cytokines, chemokines, growth factor, and adhesion molecules occurs between the fetal trophoblastic cells and maternal endometrium.

The decidual immune cells, mainly the NK cells and T helper cells, play an important role in maintaining and moderating the immune tolerance and vascular remodeling. The other proinflammatory cytokines, chemokines, and adhesion molecules play a role in establishing the endometrial receptivity and promoting blastocyst opposition and adhesion to the endometrium. Any disruption in this immunological environment can cause fetal rejection and pregnancy loss.

Natural Killer Cells

Natural killer (NK) cells are lymphocytes that form part of the innate immune system and are found in both peripheral blood and the endometrium. It has been observed that uterine NK (uNK) cells are maximum in the implantation window and that they regulate angiogenesis. Trophoblast cells express antigens that are recognized by the receptors on uNK cells. Few studies have reported an association between high prepregnancy peripheral blood NK cells and RPL,[3] but recent prospective studies found no such association.[4-6] Beer et al. reported NK cell proportion levels of over 12% of peripheral blood mononuclear cells as the cut-off for high NK cell levels.[7] However, there is no consensus on what an abnormal NK cell test result is, and normal ranges vary in different studies.

Various other studies have tried to find an association between RPL and NK cells in endometrial biopsy, however no convincing conclusions have been yet established. Thus, more advanced researches are needed before measurement of uNK cells can be recommended in routine clinical practice as an investigation for RPL.

Cytokine-mediated Immunity

Maternal immune tolerance to pregnancy is characterized by predominant induction of T-helper 2 cells and production of anti-inflammatory cytokines mainly interleukin 4, 6, and 10. The T-helper 1 cytokine response is characterized by the production of proinflammatory cytokines like interleukin 2, interferon, and TNF-α. The Th-2 type cytokine response allows the production of blocking antibodies which mask fetal trophoblast antigens from immunologic recognition by maternal Th-1 cell-mediated cytotoxic response. Disruption of T-helper cell balance in the endometrium can cause implantation failure and pregnancy loss.[8] An association between TGF-α1 and TNF-α gene polymorphisms and RPL has also been suggested.

■ IMMUNOTHERAPY IN RECURRENT PREGNANCY LOSS

As immunological and inflammatory changes play a critical role in implantation and for maintenance of pregnancy, various immunomodulatory therapies have been suggested for women with RPL. These include paternal leukocyte immunizations, IVIG, intralipids, trophoblastic infusion, anti-TNF-α drugs, and G-CSF.

Leukocyte Immunotherapy in RPL

Inadequate maternal tolerance to paternal alloantigens can cause fetal rejection and pregnancy loss. Thus, it is suggested that immunizations with paternal mononuclear cells may enhance maternal recognition of paternal alloantigens and may help women with RPL.

Mowbray et al. were the first to study the usefulness of leukocyte immunotherapy (LIT) in RPL and they reported significant improvement in live birth rate (LBR).[9] Recently, two separate meta-analyses conducted by Cavalcante et al. and Liu et al. reported an improved LBR after LIT therapy in women with RPL.[10,11] However, these studies were criticized for their low quality, low patient number, and lack of consistency in the patient population selected. A recent Cochrane review does not support the use of LIT or any other kind of immunotherapy for RPL. However, the review has been criticized by many researchers as it did not consider primary and secondary RPL separately, the number of miscarriages, immunizing doses, and routes of administration also were not considered.

Intravenous Immunoglobulin in RPL

Intravenous immunoglobulins have been widely used to treat various inflammatory and autoimmune disorders and are also being prescribed for women with RPL. The IVIG possibly exerts the beneficial effects by neutralization of cytotoxic antibodies, expansion of regulatory T cells, regulation of T-helper cell balance, and reduction of NK cell number and activity.[12-14]

However, the results of IVIG treatment in women with RPL have been controversial. A review by Coulam et al. observed that IVIG by suppressing NK cell activity enhances LBR in women with RPL and elevated NK cell levels.[15] However, two recent meta-analyses failed to see any improved results.[16,17] Also, there is no standardization of the dosage regimes, frequency of administration, and duration of therapy. The high cost and possibility of adverse effects are the other concerns with IVIG treatment.

Anti-TNF-α Drugs

Tumor necrosis factor-alpha is a proinflammatory cytokine which is produced by the Th-1 cells. It is a marker of degree of inflammation and levels are reported to be high in patients with RPL. TNF-α antagonists (adalimumab) have been used for unexplained RPL. A retrospective study conducted by Winger et al. reported that addition of adalimumab and IVIG to anticoagulants improved the LBRs compared to anticoagulants alone in patients with RPL.[18] However, the data regarding this drug is limited and no prospective studies are available. Also, there are concerns about its safety in pregnancy.[19]

Granulocyte Colony Stimulating Factor

Granulocyte colony stimulating factor is a cytokine produced by the decidual cells and is found to have a positive impact on the trophoblast. It stimulates neutrophilic granulocyte proliferation and differentiation. In a randomized controlled trial (RCT) conducted by Scarpellini et al., G-CSF administration was found to significantly improve LBR in women with recurrent abortions compared to placebo.[20] Contrary to these findings, Zafardoust et al., did not find any beneficial effect of intrauterine G-CSF in women with unexplained RPL.[21] Large multicenter trials are needed before G-CSF can be recommended as a treatment modality for RPL.

Intralipids

Intralipids used for parenteral nutrition have been shown to inhibit NK cell activity and suppress proinflammatory cytokines. Dakhly et al. used 250 mL of intralipid infusion on the day of oocyte retrieval in patients with RPL with elevated peripheral blood NK cells (>12%), and observed increased ongoing pregnancy and LBRs.[22] However further appropriately powered studies need to be conducted before this can be routinely advised in clinical practice.

Corticosteroids

Synthetic corticosteroids are known to have immunosuppressive effect on NK and Th cells and so have been explored as a potential treatment for women with RPL. Prednisolone is shown to reduce the uNK cells. Though some studies showed a beneficial effect of prednisolone in women with RPL, other failed to observe any improvement in the absence of autoimmunity. Moreover, its safety in early pregnancy is also a concern.

■ CONCLUSION

Though the role of immunological factors in women the RPL is long known, appropriate cut-off value for the evaluation of these factors is not yet established and are thus not recommended in routine clinical practice. It is a real challenge and pressure for the treating physician whether to recommend these immunotherapy modalities to women with unexplained RPL, as the results so far are controversial and further large scale studies are needed to prove their efficacy and safety.

■ RECOMMENDATION FOR IMMUNOTHERAPY IN RPL (ESHRE GUIDELINES ON RPL)[23]

- Immunological screenings including HLA determination, anti-HLA antibodies, anti-HY antibodies, cytokines, cytokine polymorphism testing, NK cell testing are not recommended in women with RPL in clinical practice.

- No immunological biomarker except for high titer antiphospholipid antibodies, can be used for selecting couples with RPL for specific immunological treatments.
- There is insufficient evidence to recommend LIT, IVIG, intralipids or G-CSF as treatment of RPL.

■ REFERENCES

1. Practice committee of American Society of Assisted Reproduction. Evaluation and treatment of recurrent pregnancy loss: a committee opinion. Fertil Steril. 2012;98:1103-11.
2. Carp HA, Toder V, Torchinsky A, et al. Allogenic leucocyte immunization in women with five or more recurrent abortins. Hum Reprod. 1997;12:250-5.
3. Aoki K, Kajiura S, Matsumoto Y, et al. Pre-conceptional natural killer cell activity as a predictor of miscarriage. The Lancet. 1995;345:1340-2.
4. Emmer PM, Verrhoek M, Nelen WL, et al. Natural killer cell reactivity and HLA-G in recurrent spontaneous abortion. Transplant Proc. 1999;31:1838-40.
5. Liang P, Mo M, Li GG, et al. Comprehensive analysis of peripheral blood lymphocytes in 76 women with recurrent miscarriage before and after lymphocyte immunotherapy. Am J Reprod Immunol. 2012;68:164-74.
6. Katano K, Suzuki S, Ozaki Y, et al. Peripheral natural killer cell activity as a predictor of recurrent pregnancy loss: a large cohort study. Fertil Steril. 2013;100:1629-34.
7. Beer AE, Kwak JY, Ruiz JE. Immunophenotypic profiles of peripheral blood lymphocytes in women with recurrent pregnancy losses and in infertile women with multiple failed in vitro fertilization cycles. Am J Reprod Immunol. 1996;35:376-82.
8. Shimada S, Kato EH, Morikawa M, et al. No difference in natural killer or natural killer T-cell population but aberrant T-helper cell population in the endometrium of women with repeated miscarriage. Hum Reprod. 2004;19:1018-24.
9. Mowbray JF, Gibben C, Udden H, et al. Controlled trial of treatment of recurrent spontaneous abortions by immunisation with paternal cells. Lancet. 1985;1: 941-3.
10. Liu Z, Xu H, Kang X, et al. Allogenic lymphocyte immunotherapy for unexplained recurrent spontaneous abortions. A meta-analysis. Am J Reprod Immunol. 2016;76:443-53.
11. Cavalcante MB, Sarno M, Araujo Junior, et al. Lymphocyte immunotherapy for the treatment of recurrent miscarraiges: systematic review and meta-analysis. Arch Gynecol Obstet. 2017;295:511-8.
12. Morikawa M, Yamada H, Kato EH, et al. Massive intravenous immunoglobulin treatment in women with four or more recurrent spontaneous abortions of unexplained etiology: down regulation of NK cell activity and subsets. Am J Reprod Immunol. 2001;46:399-404.
13. Kim DJ, Lee SK, Kim JY, et al. Intravenous immunoglobulin G modulates peripheral blood Th17 and Foxp3(+) regulatory T cells in pregnant women with recurrent pregnancy loss. Am J Reprod Immunol. 2014;71:441-50.

14. Clark DA, Wong K, Banwatt D, et al. CD 200 dependent and non-CD 200 dependent pathways of NK cell suppression by human IVIG. J Assist Reprod Genet. 2008;25:67-72.
15. Coulam CB, Acacia B. Does immunotherapy for treatment of reproductive failure enhances live births? Am J Reprod Immunol. 2012;67:296-303.
16. Rasmark Roepke E, Hellgren M, Hjertberg R, et al. Treatment efficacy for idiopathic recurrent pregnancy loss—a systematic review and meta-analyses. Acta Obstet Gynecol Scand. 2018;97:921-41.
17. Egerup P, Lindschou J, Gludd C, et al. The effects of intravenous immunoglobulin in women with recurrent miscarriages: a systematic review of randomised trials with meta-analyses and trial sequential analyses including individual patient data. PLos ONE. 2015;10:e0141588.
18. Winger EE, Reed JL. Treatment with tumor necrosis factor inhibitors and intravenous immunoglobulin improves live birth rates in women with recurrent spontaneous abortions. Am J Reprod Immunol. 2008;60:8-16.
19. Weber-Schoendorfer C, Oppermann M, Wacker E, et al. Pregnancy outcome after TNF-alpha inhibitor therapy during the first trimester: a prospective multicentre cohort study. Br J Clin Pharmacol. 2015;80:727-39.
20. Scarpellini F, Sbracia M. Use of granulocyte colony stimulating factor for the treatment of unexplained recurrent miscarriage: a randomised controlled trial. Hum Reprod. 2009;24:2703-8.
21. Zafardoust S, Akhondi MM, Sadeghi MR, et al. Efficacy of intrauterine granulocyte colony stimulating factor (G-CSF) on treatment of unexplained recurrent miscarriage: a pilot RCT study. J Reprod Infertil. 2017;18:379-85.
22. Dakhly DM, Bayoumi YA, Sharkawy M et al. intralipid supplementation in women with recurrent spontaneous abortion and elevated levels of natural killer cells. Int J Gynecol Obstet. 2016;135:324-7.
23. The ESHRE guideline group on RPL; Atik RB, Christiansen OB, Elson J, et al. ESHRE guideline: Recurrent pregnancy loss. Hum Reprod Open. 2018;1-12.

Chapter 17: Tender Loving Care

Jayam Kannan, P Prashitha

"Be healing with your words, be tender with your words, be gentle with your words and watch your words bring gentle, tender healing in the hearts of others."

—**Heather Wolf, Kipnuk Visits Sea Isle**

■ INTRODUCTION

Wherever medical care becomes incapacitated, tender loving care works miracles. Same has been officially acknowledged in the field of medicine. Doctor–patient communication, emotional support, and day-to-day life planning are becoming equally important as the right medication for recovery from illness.

Pregnancy loss can be emotionally and physically challenging for couples that too when faced repeatedly. There are numerous known causes for recurrent pregnancy loss (RPL), like anatomic, genetic, infectious, endocrine, immunologic of which 40–50% are of unknown etiology.[1] At present, there is insufficient evidence for any specific treatment for idiopathic RPL.[2] There is no definite cause in half of these patients except reassurance and tender loving care.[3]

Pregnancy loss is a significant negative life event. The psychological impact of abortion is as significant as that of stillbirth and neonatal death causing depression and anxiety for several months.[4] Studies have shown that stress increases abortive cytokine tumor necrosis factor-alpha (TGF-α) and reduces cytokine TGF-P2 which is of proimplantive nature.[5] Evidence on psychoneuroimmunological cause of RPL prove that guilt, distress, and grief cause altered levels of cortisol, CD3 +, CD56+, CD8 +, T cells, Th2 and Th1 helper cells, and NK cell activity which affect the fate of pregnancy.[6]

Women with recurrent miscarriage along with loss of pregnancy experience loss of hope, health, and self-esteem which leads to a complex grieving process.[7] Because of possible loss of fetus, there is tremendous amount of fear experienced in the following pregnancy. This fear exists even after they pass the prior miscarriage week and even postpartum.

Guidelines recommended for treatment of RPL suggest tender loving care as an approach which includes frequent counseling, psychological support, and examination to reassure the continuation of pregnancy.[8] There is five times higher incidence of moderate-to-severe depression in women having RPL than in women trying to conceive naturally. A depression prevalence of 8.6% and a high stress level in 42.1% of newly referred patients with RPL are clinically relevant. This has been evidenced by the Copenhagen study. The standard of care for patients with RPL is "tender loving care", an approach which sometimes even entails frequent ultrasound examinations in early pregnancy and psychological support, although empirical evidence for this ultrasound examination is sparse. However, evaluation of mental distress at referral is not customary in RPL clinics, as far as we know. Women with RPL may have a need for psychological counseling, also when not pregnant.

Tender loving care is one of the common and accepted treatments especially in idiopathic RPL.[9] It significantly improves the chance of live birth rate.[10] These women experience higher degree of satisfaction when their partners support them. There are few studies about men experiencing psychological stress after abortion. Hence, the couples and not only women should be involved in counseling, and discussed about risks, benefits, and alternatives of medications and treatment during preconception and pregnancy. Women who received specific counseling and support had a pregnancy success rate of 86% compared to 33% who did not receive counseling and support.[10]

A national survey that provides insight into public perceptions of the incidence and causes of miscarriage and builds on prior work looking at the emotional effects of miscarriage has been carried out in USA.[11] Those who had suffered a miscarriage frequently felt guilty, isolated, and alone. Identifying a potential cause of the miscarriage may have an effect on patients' psychological and emotional responses. About 45% alone felt comfortable with the adequate emotional support from the medical community, 25% reporting they did not receive adequate support. ESHRE guidelines clearly state that with or without specific treatment, couples value a plan for the pregnancy after RPL, with the care of a dedicated and supportive individual physician or team. There is only limited and weak evidence that this approach in itself improves pregnancy outcome, but even if not, it is hard to argue against this approach.[12]

Tender loving care does miracles, when there is no exact medical care. It has been well acknowledged in our field. Along with right diagnosis and medication, doctor–patient relation, proper communication, emotional support, and daily life planning helps the patients to overcome the stress of RPL and have a fruitful pregnancy.

CONCLUSION

"May the Lord grant you tender kind heart."

—Lailah Gifty Akita, Pearls of Wisdom: Great mind

Having a tender and kind heart is imperative in the management of couples suffering recurrent pregnancy losses. There should not be any haste in taking decisions. The couple should be provided the best care in the kindest way possible for a fruitful outcome.

REFERENCES

1. Arora M, Mukhopadhaya N. Recurrent pregnancy loss. Jaypee Brothers Medical Publishers (P) Ltd; 2018 Jun 30.
2. Roepke ER, Hellgren M, Hjertberg R, et al. Treatment efficacy for idiopathic recurrent pregnancy loss: a systematic review and meta-analyses. Acta Obstet Gynecol Scand. 2018;97:921-41.
3. Li TC. Recurrent miscarriage: Principles of management. Hum Reprod. 1998;13(2):478-82.
4. Kagami M, Maruguana T, Koizumi T, et al. Psychological adjustment and psychosocial stress among Japanese couples with a history of recurrent pregnancy loss. Hum Reprod. 2012;27(3):787-94.
5. Craig M. Stress and recurrent miscarriage. Stress. 2001;4(3):205-13.
6. Patel A, Dinesh N, Sharma PSVN, et al. Outcomes of structured psychotherapy for emotional adjustment in a childless couple diagnosed with recurrent pregnancy loss: A unique investigation. J Hum Reprod Sci. 2018;11(2):202-7.
7. Hada K, Kuse E, Nakatsuka M. Women with recurrent pregnancy loss: Their Psychology during late pregnancy and the supportive behaviour of their partners. Acta Med Okayana. 2018;72(4):387-94.
8. Kolte AM, Olser LR, Mikkelser EM, et al. Depression and emotional stress is highly prevalent among women with recurrent pregnancy loss. Hum Reprod. 2015;30(4):777-82.
9. Lachmi- Epstein A, Mazor M, Bashiri A. Psychological and mental aspects and "tender loving care" among women with recurrent pregnancy losses. Harenquah. 2012;151(11):633-7.
10. Jauriaux E, Farquharson RG, Christiansen OB, et al. Evidence-based guidelines for the investigation and medical treatment of recurrent miscarriage. Hum Reprod. 2006;21(9):2216-22.
11. Bardos J, Hercz D, Friedenthal J, et al A national survey on public perception of miscarriage. Obstet Gynecol. 2015;125(6):1313-20.
12. ESHRE guideline: Recurrent pregnancy loss. Human Reprod Open; 2018. pp. 1-12.

Index

Page numbers followed by *f* refer to figure, *fc* refer to flowchart, and *t* refer to table.

A

Abdominal cerclage, indications of 78
Acquired immune deficiency
    syndrome 111
Acquired uterine anomalies 89
Adalimumab 138
Addison's disease 19
Adenomas 99
Adenomyosis 103*f*
Adrenal hyperplasia 19
American College of Obstetricians and
    Gynecologists 75
American Society for Reproductive
    Medicine 37, 82
And anti-beta-2 glycoprotein I
    antibody 45
Androgens 10
Androstenedione 39, 66
Aneuploidy 13
    pregnancy 130
Anti-beta 2-glycoprotein I antibodies
    47, 51
Anticardiolipin antibodies 45, 46, 51
Anticoagulation therapy 53
Anti-HLA antibodies 9
Anti-HY antibodies 9
Anti-Müllerian hormone, low 19
Antinuclear antibodies 9, 48
Antiphospholipid 24, 45
Antiphospholipid antibodies
    clinical criteria 46
    clinical features 48
    complications 49
    differential diagnoses 50
    epidemiology 45
    etiology 47
    histology 52
    imaging 51
    investigations 50
    laboratory criteria 46
    pathophysiology 48
    risk factors 47
    treatment 52
Antiphospholipid antibody
    syndrome 15, 136
Antiphospholipid syndrome 3, 16, 45
    primary 18
    secondary 19
Antisperm antibodies 9, 107
Anti-thrombin deficiency 12
Antithyroid drugs propylthiouracil 63
Array-based comparative genomic
    hybridization 13
Asherman's syndrome 10, 92
Aspirin 24
Assisted reproductive technology 23,
    120
Autoimmune disorders 129
Autoimmune hemolytic anemia 49
Autoimmune thrombocytopenia 45, 49

B

Bacterial vaginosis 112
Beta-hCG 6
Bicornuate uteri 10, 31*f*, 33, 81, 87
Bicornuate uterus 34*f*
    three-dimensional image 34*f*
    two-dimensional image 34*f*
Blastocyst receptive 38
Brucellosis 19

C

Catastrophic antiphospholipid
    syndrome 45
Celiac disease serum markers 9
Cervical cerclage, methods of 76

Cervical encerclage, principal of 75
Cervical factors in
   cervical incompetence 73
   contributory 72
   diagnosis 73
   etiopathogenesis 73
   management 75
   postoperative care/concerns 78
Cervical incompetence 19
   evaluation 74
   examination5 74
Cervical insufficiency 73
Chlamydia 111
Chlamydia trachomatis 11, 110, 114
Chorea gravidarum 49
Chorionic gonadotropin receptor 38
Chromosomal
   abnormalities 105
   microdeletions 105
Cold-knife technique 97
Collin's knife 93
Comparative genome hybridization 120, 132
Conception, implantation 61
Conception, products of 24
Connective tissue synechiae 94
Corpus luteum 38
Corticosteroids 139
Coxsackie virus 110
Cytogenetic abnormalities 136
Cytokine-mediated immunity 137
Cytokines 9
Cytomegalovirus 110

D

De novo during embryogenesis 21
Density lipoprotein
   intermediate 63
   low 63
Diabetes mellitus 67
Didelphic uterus 81
Diethylstilbestrol in utero 73
Dioscorea mexicana 38
Dioscorea tokoro 38
Disseminated intravascular coagulation 50
DNA fragmentation index 6, 131
Dydrogesterone 40, 42

E

Ectopic pregnancy 2
Embryonic
   aneuploidies 129
   miscarriage 2
Endocrine dysfunction 68
Endocrine Society Clinical Practice Guideline 63
Endometrial
   fibrosis 92
   function test 43
   polyp 28*f*, 100*f*
Endometritis: chronic, treatment of 114
Endometrium 98
Enoxaparin 58
Enterobacter 111
Enterococcus 114
Enzyme-linked immunosorbent assay 51
Epigenetics 106
Epitope mimicry in autoimmune disease 48
Escherichia coli 114
Espinosa-flores operation 77, 77*f*
Estradiol valerate, cycles of 87
Estrogen-primed proliferative endometrium 38
Estrone by aromatase 39
Euploid 13
European Society for Gynaecological Endoscopy 82
European Society for Human Reproduction and Embryology 9, 37, 82

F

False-positive serologic test 49
Fetal deaths 50
Fetal fibronectin 74
Fetal genomics 13
Fetal growth restriction 45
Fetal loss 45, 49
Fetal Medicine Foundation 27
Fetal miscarriage 2
Fetal trisomy 18
Fibroids 26, 95
   standard procedure 96

Index

Filmy adhesions 96*f*
Fluorescence in situ hybridization 13, 21, 105, 132
Folic acid, role of 66
Follicle biosynthesize 38
Follicle-stimulating hormone receptor 39
Fragile endometrial synechiae 93
Free androgen index 66
Free radical attack 106

G

Gardnerella vaginalis 111, 114
Genetic
    abnormalities, source of 21
    causes 12, 13
    miscarriages, hallmark of 20
    techniques 13
    tests
        advantages of 22
        modalities of 21
    thrombophilic factors 12
    bacterial vaginosis 19
Genital tuberculosis 112
Genome hybridization 106
Global Antiphospholipid Syndrome Score 51
Glycosaminoglycan 73
Gonadotropin-releasing hormone use of 39
Granulocyte colony stimulating factor 136, 138
Granulosa cells 38, 39
Graves' disease 9

H

Haemophilus influenzae 48
Hemorrhagic cysts 103*f*
Heparin
    mode of action 57
    use of
        antiphospholipid syndrome 58
        hereditary thrombophilia 58
        thrombosis 58
Herpes simplex virus 11, 110
Heterotrisomy 129
Hormonal and metabolic disorders 136

HOXA10 gene 66
Human chorionic gonadotropin 2
Human leukocyte antigen 8, 48, 136
Human reproduction 72, 118
Human spermatozoa 106
Hyaluronic acid 73
Hyperandrogenemia 61, 65, 66
Hyperandrogenism 19
Hyperhomocysteinemia 10, 19, 61, 66
Hyperinsulinemia 65
Hyperprolactinemia 19, 61, 66
Hyperthyroidism 9, 63
    subclinical 62
Hysterosalpingogram 24, 83
Hysteroscopic polypectomy 101*f*

I

Immunological tests 9
In vitro fertilization 23, 39, 129
Inflammatory autoimmune diseases 52
Inherited thrombophilias 136
Inherited thrombophilias, testing of 14
Insulin resistance 61, 65
Intracytoplasmic sperm injection 23, 131
Intralipids 139
Intramural fibroids 10
Intrauterine adhesions 28, 90
    band of 95*f*
    prevention of 87
    standard procedure 93
Intrauterine growth restriction 81
Intrauterine pathologies 80

K

Klebsiella pneumoniae 114

L

Labor and delivery, management of 54
Landry-Guillain-Barré-Strohl syndrome 49
Leukocyte immunotherapy 138
Levothyroxine 63
Listeria and intracellular bacteria 112
Listeria monocytogenes 110
Live birth rate 138

Livedo reticularis 49
Loop electrode 99
Lupus anticoagulant 24, 45, 47, 50
Luteal phase defects 19
Luteal phase
   deficiency 61, 66
   insufficiency 10
Luteinizing hormone 10
   hypersecretion of 61, 65
Lyme's disease 19

M

Male factors 11
Male urogenital infections 19
Maternal dietary iodine deficiency 61
Maternal obesity 65
Maternofetal alloimmune response 136
McDonald operation 76, 76*f*
Metabolic and endocrinologic factors 9
Methimazole 63
Methylenetetrahydrofolate reductase mutation 12
Methyltetrahydrofolate gene homozygosity 19
Micronized progesterone 42
Molecular weight heparin, low 56, 66
Monosomy X 118
Müllerian
   abnormalities 19
   anomalies 10
Multiorgan failure 50
Mycoplasma 11, 110, 113
Mycoplasma hominis 114
Myofibrous synechiae 93
Myoma, resection of 98*f*, 99

N

Natural killer cells 9, 137
Neisseria gonorrhoeae 48, 114
Neisseria meningitidis 50
Neonatal lupus dermatitis 50
Next-generation sequencing 22, 120, 132

O

Obesity 61, 65
Obstetric care 52

Office hysteroscopy 85
Oocyte retrieval 40
Ovarian reserve testing 10
Overt hypothyroidism 62

P

Paracentric 130
Parental genetic analysis 14
Parental karyotyping 22
Paternal leukocyte immunization 136
Pericentric inversions 130
Perinatal morbidity 50
Pituitary thyroid-stimulating hormone 61
Plasminogen activator inhibitor 19
Polycystic ovarian syndrome 10, 19, 65
Polymerase chain reaction 114, 132
Polypectomy forceps 101*f*
Polyploidy 18
Polypoidal adenomyoma 102*f*
Polyps 10, 98
Preeclampsia, thrombosis 45
Pregnancy loss 142
   biochemical 2
   clinical 3
   early 2, 37
   late 2
   preclinical 3
   terminology 4
   very early 6
Pregnenolone diffuses 38
Preimplantation genetic
   diagnosis 14, 23, 24, 118, 119, 132
      in carriers of balanced translocation 132
   screening 14, 22-24, 119, 121, 129
      unexplained recurrent pregnancy loss 132
   testing 118
Preterm premature rupture of membranes 74
Progesterone 40
   early pregnancy trial of 43
   history of 38
   in menstrual cycle 38
   in ovarian cycle 38, 39*f*
   luteal phase support 39

Index

production triggers 67
role of 39
therapy 44
use of 42
Proinflammatory cytokine 138
Prolactin 10, 12
Prothrombin
  gene mutation 19
  mutation 12

R

Recurrent implantation failure 6
Recurrent miscarriage 1
  causes of 18
  clinical trial 2*t*
  etiology of 20*f*
Recurrent pregnancy loss 1, 56
  access to care 124
  anatomical
    causes of 80
    investigation 10
  antiphospholipids in 45
  application and acceptance in 118
  cervical factors in 72
  clinic 124
    assessment of couple 125
    dissemination of knowledge 125
    equipment 125
    first visit 125
    location 125
    personnel needed 124
    planning and approach 126
    psychological counseling 126
    research 126
  cytogenetic abnormality 129
  DNA
    damage 106
    fragmentation 130
  due to
    environmental toxins 106
    oxidative stress 106
  endocrinological perspectives in 61
  environmental etiologies 11
  etiology of 8*f*, 105
  genetic
    causes of 18
    factors in 118
  guidelines 1, 4
  heparin in 56
  hysteroscopy in 80
  hysterosonography 28
  immunological screening 8
  immunotherapy in 136, 137, 139
  indications for ART in 23
  infections 110-115
    antibiotics in unexplained 115
    chronic endometritis 113
    etiologies 11
    massive chronic intervillositis 114
    pathogenesis 111
    treatment in 115
  international guidelines 42
  intravenous immunoglobulin in 138
  investigations in 8
  leukocyte immunotherapy in 137
  major endocrinological causes of 61
  male contribution to 130
  organisms contributing to 110
  paternal age 107
  preimplantation genetic
    diagnosis 131
    screening 131
    testing for 118, 120
  progesterone, hormone 37
  promise study 41
  role of
    assisted reproduction in 129
    male factor in 105
    progesterone 40
    seminal fluid in 107
    surrogacy in 133
    ultrasound in 26
  setting up clinic 124
  strategy for management of couples 127
  three-dimensional ultrasound 29
  transvaginal ultrasound 26
  treatment options 22
  unexplained 14, 120
  workup for early 24*fc*
Recurrent spontaneous miscarriage 37
Renal system abnormalities 81
Resectoscope 85
Respiratory distress syndrome 115
Rett syndrome 18

Robertsonian 130
Robertsonian translocations 118, 119
Royal College of Obstetricians and
    Gynaecologists 37
Rubella 110
Rudimentary horn 87

S

Seminal fluid 107
Septate and bicornuate uterus 35*t*
Septate uterus 19, 81, 82*f*
    classification 82
    complete 84*f*
    diagnosis 82
    hysterosalpingography 83*f*
    methods of surgical treatment 85
    ultrasonography 83*f*
Septum
    resection of 86*f*
    with resectoscope resection of 86*f*
Serum hCG levels, low 61, 67
Serum pregnancy test 40
Shigella dysenteriae 48
Shirodkar operation 76, 77*f*
Single-nucleotide polymorphism array
    21, 132
Sperm
    aneuploidy 105, 131
    donation 132
    quality 11
Spontaneous abortion 81
Spontaneous pregnancy loss 8, 15
Staphylococcus 114
Submucosal fibroids 10
Subseptate uterus 84*f*
Syphilis 112
    systemic 19

T

Tender loving care 142, 143
Testosterone 66
Th-1 cells 138
Theca cells 38
Thrombophilia 12, 129

Thrombotic thrombocytopenic
    purpura 50
Thyroglobulin 64
    antibody, incidence of 62
Thyroid autoantibodies 10
Thyroid autoimmunity 64
Thyroid disease 61
Thyroid dysfunction 9, 61
    in pregnancy 64*fc*
Thyroid hormone, normal levels of 62
Thyroid peroxidase antibody 62
Thyroid-stimulating hormone 24, 64
Toxoplasma gondii 110
Toxoplasmosis 19
Trisomy 118
Trophectoderm 23
Trophoblastic infusions 136
Tuberculosis 112
Tumor necrosis factor-alpha 138, 142

U

Unicornuate uterus 10, 81, 87, 88*f*, 89*f*
    class II 90*f*
    hysteroscopic view of 92*f*
Ureaplasma 11, 110
Uterine anomalies 26, 80, 81, 129, 136
    congenital 81
    ESHRE/ESGE classification of 31*f*
    prevalence of 81*t*
Uterine cavity 28
    normal 84*f*
Uterine fibroids 10
Uterine septum 10, 19, 82

V

Vaginal micronized progesterone 40, 42
Villous thrombosis 65

W

Waterhouse-Friderichsen syndrome 50
Wurm operation 77, 77*f*

Y

Y chromosomal microdeletions 19
Yolk sac miscarriage 2

www.ingramcontent.com/pod-product-compliance
Ingram Content Group UK Ltd.
Pitfield, Milton Keynes, MK11 3LW, UK
UKHW051902120525
458461UK00003B/13